Since developing multiple sclerosis well over 15 years ago, Cynthia Benz has experienced many of its ups and downs. She has had first-hand experience of how incapacitating MS can be. She also knows what it is like to be freed again from its grip, with stick, wheelchair or scooter stored away once more.

Her first early enforced retirement was broken by a return to full-time work and play! In her professional life she has worked as a lecturer in adult education and as a counsellor. She has recently completed a full-time MA course and is about to begin doctoral studies. Her voluntary work includes being a trustee of the MS Society and chaplaincy visiting for a local hospital. She enjoys the good things of life to the full, especially the arts and travelling.

Cynthia has often spoken on living well with MS – at MS workshops and conferences in the British Isles and abroad, and on the radio.

She is married and lives in Berkshire.

'An acknowledgement to you,
whose love, acceptance and counsel
have made all the difference
and enabled me to walk free,
a dream come true.
My love and thanks'
                    Cynthia

COPING WITH
MULTIPLE
SCLEROSIS

A comprehensive guide to the symptoms and treatments

Cynthia Benz

Illustrated by
Shaun Williams

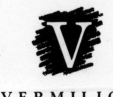

VERMILION
LONDON

First published by Macdonald Optima in 1988
Revised edition published by Optima in 1993

1 3 5 7 9 10 8 6 4 2

This edition published in the United Kingdom in 1996 by Vermilion, an imprint of Ebury Press

Random House UK Ltd
Random House
20 Vauxhall Bridge Road
London SW1V 2SA

Random House Australia (Pty) Ltd
20 Alfred Street
Milsons Point, Sydney
New South Wales 2016, Australia

Random House New Zealand Limited
18 Poland Road, Glenfield
Auckland 10, New Zealand

Random House South Africa (Pty) Limited
PO Box 337, Bergvlei, South Africa

Random House UK Limited Reg. No. 954009

A CIP catalogue record for this book is available from the British Library.

ISBN 0 09 181361 1

Typeset by Deltatype Ltd, Birkenhead, Merseyside
Printed and bound in Great Britain by Mackays of Chatham, plc

Papers used by Vermilion are natural, recyclable products made from wood grown in sustainable forests.

CONTENTS

FOREWORD

In the week you read this, about 50 other people will have been diagnosed with Multiple Sclerosis in Britain. *You are not alone.* Cynthia Benz distils in this book her own experience and that of many other people who have found their own paths to coming to terms with MS. For some people, MS is the greatest catastrophe imaginable; for others it is a recurring inconvenience. MS may produce no measurable symptoms during one person's life, while in another's it can cause severe and obvious disability and distress. The way a person copes with MS has little to do with how severe their symptoms are. Here you have an idea of the uncertainty that is virtually the only common feature of this baffling and unpredictable disorder of the central nervous system.

For almost everyone, MS is not simply a disease defined by their doctor; instead it is something that permeates many aspects – perhaps every corner – of their lives in unexpected and subtle ways. Coping successfully with MS is rarely just a matter of accepting the diagnosis and getting on with life. It may call for physical adjustments, but adaptations in emotional, personal and social life may be far more important. Cynthia Benz describes in graphic but undramatic terms the changes in way of life and habits of mind that can help everyone affected by MS, whether directly suffering from it, or suffering from the effects of it in someone close to them. As she says, 'Feelings . . . exist like toes or fingers as a natural part of you.'

This is the special character of this remarkable book; others deal with the physical facts or the psychological impact of MS; here we consider the whole person without preaching a particular philosophy or lifestyle, neither overdramatizing nor underplaying the condition and what it may mean for the individual. Since the first edition was published, treatments for the underlying disease have begun to emerge, but even so a radical cure is not yet in sight.

For the foreseeable future, the person with MS will continue to be the expert in managing and living with this strange condition. This unassuming volume is packed with wisdom and understanding of how to develop and use that expertise. It is an extraordinary testimony to human resilience, the triumph of intellect and spirit over a disorder that has defied medical science and technology for more than 150 years.

Peter Cardy
Chief Executive,
Multiple Sclerosis Society of Great Britain
and Northern Ireland

1

What is
Multiple Sclerosis?

A personal definition of MS

Anyone who has ever come into contact with multiple sclerosis will already have his or her own definition of it. Its behaviour is so infuriatingly unpredictable that no two cases are ever quite alike. Its hallmark is uncertainty – it is difficult to be certain where it begins and ends. It is as if there were a kaleidoscope of symptoms on offer, each of which comes in a variety of colours and intensities. Against that is a time factor in which symptoms appear, disappear and reappear like the most intricate movements of a bizarre dance that you have never seen before, the patterns and rhythms of which you are just getting used to when it changes totally to a haphazard jumble. MS is not easy to define simply; it revels in being elusive and difficult to catch hold of.

It helps to learn what MS can be like and what to expect. The more information you have about it, the easier it is to understand and accept. It is also important to be clear about what MS is not. It has nothing at all to do with mental disorders or so-called nervous breakdowns. It is not something you can catch like an infection. Nor is it strictly hereditary – there is no clear pattern of inheritance – although recent research does indicate that as in the development of other diseases, one factor appears to be a genetic susceptibility towards MS. Your personal definition of MS must take account of these facts.

If you have multiple sclerosis, you have the right to your own definition of MS, and the right to keep that definition open, changing it as you need to. You will meet many people who are sure they know what MS is. They may try to convince you that you are typical, atypical, better or worse off than the standard, average person with MS – they seem to know so much about it. You have the right to be yourself and to experience your MS your way.

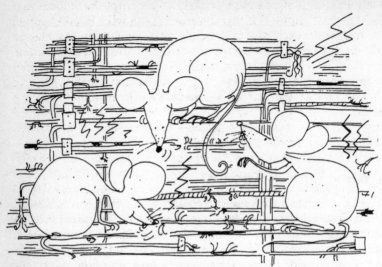

.. THE EFFECT OF AN ATTACK ON THE MYELIN SHEATH CAN
BE COMPARED TO THAT OF MICE NIBBLING AT THE
INSULATION AROUND WIRES IN A TELEPHONE EXCHANGE ...

A clinical definition of MS

Multiple sclerosis is an inflammatory demyelinating condition, one
of the most common diseases of the central nervous system, or
CNS. The cause of multiple sclerosis still remains unknown. It is
rather like a giant jigsaw puzzle with thousands of researchers, all
experts in various branches of science, painstakingly putting
together the pieces they recognize and trying to add in other pieces
that look like a promising fit. What is known about MS is that
myelin, a fatty sheath insulating the nerves, is damaged and lost, a
process known as *demyelination*. Myelin enables nerves to conduct
electrical impulses swiftly to and from the brain. The loss of myelin
disrupts and slows down the normal smooth working of the nerves.
This disruption is responsible for producing the various symptoms
of MS. Scars develop, a process known as *sclerosis*, at the sites where
the myelin is lost. It is more usual to refer to the scars as *plaques* or
lesions. Because there are so many areas of sclerosis in MS, the
disease has been given a name that describes what can be seen in
the brain or spinal cord – *multiple sclerosis* or literally 'many scars'.
MS was formerly known as disseminated sclerosis for the same
reason, because the sclerosis was scattered in the CNS.

It is easy enough to understand how an attack on the myelin

sheath and resulting damage is likely to interrupt the smooth and steady flow of impulses if you compare it with what would happen in a telephone exchange if a family of mice got in and started nibbling the insulating material around the wires. There would be shorts and telephone calls just would not get through. In the CNS it is demyelination that causes either distortion or blocking of messages. Either they are never transmitted to their target in the first place, they go astray completely, or they are modified or slowed down *en route*. MS symptoms are the visible signs of what happens when myelin is damaged.

The central nervous system is one part the body we tend to take for granted but it will be useful at this point to outline the role it plays. It operates as the body's nerve control centre and consists of the brain, the spinal cord running down the length of the backbone, and the optic nerves. The CNS links up with the peripheral nervous system and its impulses control co-ordination, and all movements, voluntary and involuntary. Information is also fed back to the CNS from muscles and sensory organs. Each time you pick up a cup, play a musical instrument or drive a vehicle, you are dependent on the smooth functioning of the CNS to be able to carry out such complex and skilled operations.

The messages transmitted via the CNS from the brain to the body, or from the body to the brain, affect various nerves: sensory nerves, to do with feeling; motor, to do with movement; and optic, to do with seeing. Because they travel at very high speeds, you experience the transmission of the messages as instantaneous. It is a highly efficient body system that never takes a break even when you are asleep. So what happens if there is some blockage or interference in a nerve pathway, the result of the interference caused by demyelination, is the sort of knock-on effect that is experienced with MS.

In order to discuss demyelination, however simply, it helps to know first something about the way nerve cells normally function. The nerve cell, or neurone, billions of which together form what we know as 'grey matter', is the basic unit of the CNS. Each nerve cell has a nerve fibre, or axon, leading from it. Axons are like pathways, making connections with other nerve cells, in muscles and sensory organs such as your ears, eyes and skin, and with internal organs like the heart or stomach. They are fine and delicate and can be very long – as in the spinal cord – or short, as in the brain, where compactness is crucial. Because their role in transmitting messages is so vital, they are protected by layers of specialized cells called *oligodendrocytes*, which wrap themselves round axons like a coating and enable rapid transmissions of impulses. This protective layer is known as the *myelin sheath*. Myelin is made up of lipids and proteins in a complex chemical substance that insulates. Because of its colour it is sometimes referred to as the 'white matter' of the brain and spinal cord. A healthy axon with its protective myelin sheath undamaged is supplied with nutrients by cells called *astrocytes*.

Inflammation of and damage to the myelin sheath (demyelination) are the root causes of MS. How this happens is not certain but it is thought to be a result of healthy tissue being damaged by the immune system. Since the CNS is the most vital control module in the body, any damage to it has serious consequences. In fact, the CNS has a unique and specialized system of protection to safeguard its function. This is called the *blood-brain barrier* and it works as a sort of filter, keeping a close check on what substances enter the CNS. The blood-brain barrier works in conjunction with the body's own immune system, which exists to protect the body against attack by viruses, bacteria or other foreign material. An additional protection in the brain and spinal cord is its supply of special fluid, *cerebrospinal* fluid, or CSF. This bathes the nerve tissue and an adequate quantity of it is needed to ensure balanced function. Analysis of CSF using samples obtained by a lumbar puncture may point to an MS diagnosis.

Thus the immune system and the unique protective systems of the CNS are on stand-by in case of attack. With MS the attack is *against* parts of the myelin sheath and the CNS responds by showing signs of inflammation. Once attacked, the body responds by increasing its production of white blood cells (lymphocytes) and there is a concurrent increase in fluid, or *oedema*. When the attack has been dealt with, the inflammation dies down. The myelin that was under attack may now heal up completely or may continue to show signs of damage. Myelinated axons can transmit nerve impulses up to ten times faster than unmyelinated axons. Many MS symptoms are attributable to poor conduction, caused by damage to the myelin.

Although it is not known for sure why the myelin sheath breaks down, it is thought possible that minimal breakdowns are normal for everyone. It would follow that most bodies either tolerate such minor damage and/or that some remyelination is a normal response. It is further speculated that some people may have *poor quality* myelin which spontaneously breaks down before it could be aggravated or precipitated by other factors such as a highly localized auto-immune reaction.

Each sclerosis or lesion has the potential to interfere with the transmission of impulses along the nerve pathways. It is possible that a single lesion can cause symptoms of MS, especially the early ones. However, a diagnosis of MS can only be made when a doctor is convinced that there is evidence of multiple scarring of tissue and that is when he or she can pick out recurring symptoms from different parts of the CNS over a period of time. Not all lesions produce obvious symptoms, however. Detailed scans sometimes reveal surprisingly large areas of sclerosis even though there have been no symptoms evident. On the other hand, just a few lesions in a couple of key places can cause a lot of havoc.

How the immune system works is incompletely understood. However, what is known is that via a complex process it identifies foreign materials, viruses, bacteria and antigens, and destroys them. Normally, the immune system is able to differentiate between healthy body tissue (*self*) and invaders (*non-self*). However, with MS it is thought that the immune system behaves abnormally and attacks healthy tissue. That is why MS is described as predominantly an *auto-immune disease.* The theoretical model of how this might happen suggests that the immune system gets its plasma cells, macrophages, lymphocytes and reactive astrocytes to attack the myelin sheath. It seems rather like having a faithful, tireless protector change character completely and run amok, hell-bent on destruction.

No one can be certain what causes the immune system to attack myelin, but it seems likely to be a combination of several factors. One theory is that a viral agent may play a key role in the development of MS. The virus might already be lying dormant in the body and be activated to trouble the immune system. Alternatively by some indirect means the virus might set off the auto-immune process. Although there is no evidence of a specific MS virus, a common virus such as measles or herpes may trigger the auto-immune process. Whatever the trigger, it activates the lymphocytes in the bloodstream and they get through the blood-brain barrier into the brain. There they apparently join forces with other elements of the immune system to attack and destroy myelin. In response to the damage, lesions are formed at the point of attack. The areas of lesion show up clearly on magnetic resonance imaging (MRI) scans.

Research is being conducted and co-ordinated world-wide to find out the cause of MS. Researchers are investigating the detailed mechanics of the body's immune reactions, viral attack, the metabolic system, genetics, the effects of trauma and stress and various combinations of these. Their discoveries help towards a better understanding of MS, an improved control of the disease and its eventual cure.

Who gets MS?

If the cause of MS were known and its course fully understood, it would be possible to predict who would be likely targets of the disease. As it is, there is general agreement among neurologists that this is, as yet, impossible, despite experimental claims that special blood testing can give clear proof of susceptibility towards MS.

Nevertheless research throws up some interesting data which reveal certain patterns. Unfortunately, MS is a young person's disease. Its symptoms most often appear between late childhood and the late fifties, with a peak between 29 and 33 years. With the use of specialized diagnostic markers such as the MRI scanner, cases of MS can be definitely diagnosed before adolescence. The older you get, the smaller the risk of developing MS, although it is still possible to develop it well into the sixties in rare cases. Fifty per cent more women develop MS than men, the ratio being three to two, and they do so at a slightly earlier age.

In terms of population, the world and individual countries can be divided into high- and low-risk MS zones. The closer to the equator or the poles an area is, the fewer cases of MS there are. The temperate latitudes of between 40 and 60 degrees are the high-risk zones. In the northern hemisphere this includes the British Isles, northern and central Europe, Iceland, Canada and the northern states of the USA. In the southern hemisphere, New Zealand, Tasmania and the southern tracts of Australia are included. Children brought up in a high-risk area who later migrate to a low-risk one appear to carry with them a high susceptibility to the disease. The reverse is also true. If children have spent their early lives (pre-puberty) in a low-risk area, they do not normally develop MS. MS is definitely more common in white races than in other racial groups. It is unknown among pure-bred Bantus and Eskimos, and among Native Americans too. MS is also uncommon among the Chinese and Japanese, who have a specialized variety of the disease.

As an example of a high-risk zone, in the British Isles it is estimated that 80 persons in 100,000 suffer from MS. This figure doubles in north-east Scotland and sky-rockets to between 250 and 300 per 100,000 in the Orkney and Shetland Islands, the highest prevalence in the world. Researchers are often struck by clusters of people with MS living locally, but the only explanations for this have been statistical coincidence and the possibility that a high incidence of MS may reflect a specific susceptibility of the native population.

MS is more prevalent in areas with high standards of sanitation. It is therefore possible that lack of exposure to some immunity-building factor makes children more susceptible to MS.

Once MS is in the family, can it be passed on? This very real fear needs to be talked about openly. MS is not infectious or contagious. You cannot catch it from someone else. Nor is it inherited in the usual sense of the word. However, there is evidence to suggest a genetically determined tendency that increases susceptibility to MS. Persons with MS are very likely to share the same tissue groups and this may be associated with the immunological system – the way the body defends itself against infections. About 10 per cent of those with MS have a blood relative with it (parent, brother, sister or child). MS in parents and children is less common than MS in brothers and sisters. Studies of identical twins show that there is a significantly increased chance of developing MS than between other brothers and sisters. It is also important to note that environmental factors such as lack of oxygen at birth or more childhood infections may also predispose towards MS. For further information on these issues, please see Chapter 6.

Is there an MS personality? Any answer to that is likely to be subjective, but it is tempting to agree that there are some strong characteristics that many persons with MS seem to share. The stereotype is of an active, healthy, attractive young adult who works long, hard, unselfishly and without complaint, putting up with things rather stoically – maybe even a bit of a perfectionist.

Patterns of MS

MS in its early stages follows a fluctuating pattern with ups and downs, starts and stops. For some it is always that way. It's a bit like having an internal weather system of symptoms as changeable as a spring day of sunshine and showers. MS symptoms can last for minutes or days, or linger for weeks, months or years. They vary tremendously in intensity, and appear and reappear in different combinations. Any variation is possible. This is why MS is described as a 'remitting and relapsing' disease.

Certainly the most common early pattern of the disease is that of relapse and remission, terms which need to be understood. When MS flares up because of inflammation and demyelination in the CNS, it is known as a *relapse*. Some people refer to it as an attack or bout of MS instead. New symptoms occur or old ones you hoped had gone for ever return. This is because a new area of demyelination is developing or an old one is being extended/reactivated. A relapse can be quite mild or relatively severe and last from just a few days to a much longer period. A relapse is rarely traced to a known cause, although it's tempting to try and blame something. It may be triggered off by infection, stress or trauma. Many people are hardly surprised when a relapse appears after a prolonged period of overdoing things – fun as well as work. Sometimes it seems as if the 'flu bugs that are laying everyone else low don't come out as 'flu in a person with MS, but aggravate MS symptoms. Some prefer to call this an exacerbation rather than a relapse, since it is a more temporary form. An old symptom will appear or become exaggerated for a time – as short as minutes or as long as a few days.

A 'remission' is when the MS flare-up stops. The symptoms of the relapse subside and disappear either partially or completely for weeks, months, years or decades. A remission is what every person with MS longs for. It is amazing that there is the potential in our bodies for complete reversal of even the severest and most entrenched disability. In the 'benign' form of MS, remission is often complete even after many exacerbations, and permanent disability does not develop.

There is no set pattern of relapses and remissions, and the variations from person to person and within the course of a lifetime are infinite. Not everyone with MS is able to identify a clear-cut distinction between relapse and remission, and some fret unnecessarily as to whether they are in one or the other; it is just as common to drag along 'betwixt and between'. This no man's land is a lonely place to be. It feels like being isolated in a tunnel with no end in sight. Suddenly you can be out in the dazzling light again or you may stay in a grey world for a while. There is always an end to that tunnel. The grey area of no clear pattern of relapse and remission becomes more common for some the longer they have MS. Their symptoms settle in, and life becomes more even and predictable.

The relationship between the body and the emotions is very important in MS, not only in relapse and remission but within any given day. Mood swings are very common and perfectly understandable, because with MS you never know what to expect. Just when you think you have come to terms with one way of feeling, you get catapulted to another and adjustment starts all over again. Any CNS damage is characterized by accompanying emotional ups and downs, and this is especially true for MS. Demyelination can have a physiological effect on the emotions, either intensifying or depressing them. It is important to accept this as fact. A person with MS will sometimes feel unreasonably or inexplicably sad, angry, fearful or happy. A later section in the book will investigate how to cope with this.

The course and types of MS

Life expectancy with MS can be close to the norm. If anything life expectancy for women is statistically slightly less. However, Hilary,

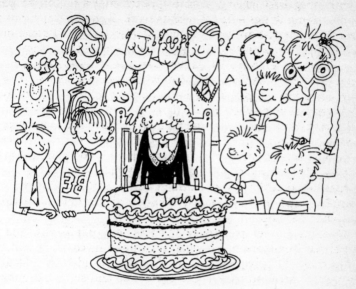

M S IS NOT NECESSARILY A DISEASE YOU DIE OF.....

now in her eighties, has had MS since her early thirties. She has two sons, and despite being in a wheelchair for over 40 years, gets out and about with the help of her caring husband. Her cheerful resilience and warmth are inspiring, as is her quality of life.

No one knows what course a particular case of MS will take. If you stand back and look at the experience of a large group of people with MS, certain patterns seem to emerge. Once you move in closer and focus on any individual, it's impossible to fit any one pattern neatly to any one person. The patterns offer general guidelines only to what is within the realm of possibility. That doesn't mean that a present trend will unfold into a future pattern. Any variation or combination is possible. MS can stop and start, reverse, and disappear.

However, from a neurological perspective, there are recognizable types of MS. Most people with MS experience it in a mild form with minimal neurological symptoms, and suffer limited and usually transitory disability. MS for them starts suddenly, may be inconvenient occasionally but is, to all intents and purposes, under control. This is a benign form of MS which often passes unnoticed by the outside world because it is mostly in a remission stage. For some, such a remission lasts a full lifetime, with permanent recovery after the first relapse. This is more likely to be so if the initial symptom is an attack of *retrobulbar neuritis* (blurred vision) followed by a long remission, or if the initial symptoms are sensory ones. For 25 per cent or so, MS runs a very benign course and no permanent disability is expected in the future. No one knows why: either the initial attack is never repeated or there is very little external evidence of demyelination. Some people live and die after a long, full, active life, with never a suspicion of MS and yet a post-mortem examination will reveal extensive areas of lesion. So in plenty of cases, MS need not disrupt the lifestyle of the individual or family, and may turn out to be a minor health hiccup.

Inevitably, though, the pattern of MS you remember and recoil from most is the one that stares at you from pictures in charity appeal literature. It tugs at your heart-strings, and rightly so, for a small proportion of people with MS (around 10 per cent) are severely afflicted with a progressive form from the start which will confine them to a wheelchair and bed. Primary progressive MS tends to start later in life, the first symptoms appearing in the mid-forties. Typical characteristics are weakness and stiffness in walking, problems with balance, slurred speech, and impaired bladder function. Sufferers are visibly disabled and need nursing care. For them, MS probably wormed its way into their lives, its physical symptoms relentlessly worsening and disability settling in permanently. This seemed to be the way Charlotte's MS was going, and with a young family of three children under five, life looked short and bleak. Then there came a halt – remission brought a reprieve – and she has since coasted along a plateau, but with clear improvements visible. Those who knew her at her lowest are amazed at her recovery against all odds. However, if MS does move into an acute crisis stage fast, it can prove fatal; thankfully, this is exceptionally uncommon.

By far the most common pattern is an abrupt onset and for the early stages of MS to be marked by relapses – either with new symptoms or with old ones intensified, each relapse followed by a gradual easing up of these symptoms. How often relapses will occur is impossible to state with any certainty. One figure much quoted is an average of one every two years, but it is possible either to go through quite a run of them in a couple of years or so, or to seem never to emerge fully from a relapse long enough to tell. Although there is no proof of what triggers an attack, it frequently seems to happen after infection. Any frequency of relapse and remission is possible.

The relapsing-remitting type of MS affects the majority of people with MS. It is the type that young adults in their twenties and thirties usually experience, with sensory symptoms like numbness, pins and needles, and tingling, weakness, stiffness and blurred vision. After the initial period, there usually follows a static stage when the pattern of relapse and remission tends to settle and symptoms stabilize. You may experience only minor exacerbations due to stress, fatigue or other factors. MS can then continue indefinitely in this long-lasting or chronic way. It may hopefully subside into remission.

The benign form of MS described above is one end of the scale of the relapsing-remitting type. The general rule of neurological thumb suggests that within the first 15 years after the symptoms of demyelination become evident, the degree of disability you experience may give something of a rough guide to your future with MS. If you are only mildly affected thus far, you are likely to remain this way. Otherwise after some years MS can flare up into acute episodes with a slow progression of permanent symptoms developing. This slow relapsing and remitting start with a more disabling continuation is the type known as the secondary progressive type of MS, which may affect up to about 40 per cent. There are, of course, exceptions either way, a fact that will not surprise you with MS!

Because MS is so unpredictable, it is important to take it a day at a time, whatever pattern or stage it seems to be in. It is understandable to panic at times at what can happen with MS, but you should never make assumptions about tomorrow on the evidence of today. If you can allow your panic to run its course without taking undue notice of it, you will find you come through. It is at times like this when people with MS long to know how everything will turn out. They think it would help to know what pattern they fit in to and what the future holds. No one can give them that information. That may be just as well, for once you fit MS too neatly into a mould, it tends to get stuck there. Christopher was permanently angry with his doctors for not being able to tell him what to expect next with MS. He came across as being aggressive, irritable, over-excited and unable to settle to living. He was so busy being upset with the unpredictability of his MS that he wasn't giving himself a chance. Do what you can gently to give your body every chance of rehabilitation whenever possible. This includes keeping your muscles supple, getting all the rest you need and want, eating a healthy diet, and keeping a positive attitude. This may seem a tall order when the going is rough, but it's one that pays dividends.

Looking at MS symptoms

The presence of symptoms, correctly verified, is proof of MS, and it is against these symptoms that the daily battle with MS is waged. Symptoms can affect the sensory areas of the body, muscles, particular organs such as the eyes or bladder, functions controlled by the central nervous system and general co-ordination. Individual symptoms result from demyelination in various parts of the brain and spinal cord.

When discussing symptoms, doctors will give information about MS that may at first seem to be contradictory. On the one hand, they may reassure you that you are unlikely to develop many symptoms, while on the other, they will tell you straight that MS is a disease that cannot be controlled. If MS is uncontrollable, it should follow logically that there's nothing to stop you from developing all the symptoms going. Fortunately, that is not the experience of most people with MS. MS symptoms cover a wide range, and you certainly don't have to have them all to have MS. In fact, it is highly unlikely for any individual to experience all of the possible symptoms.

For a diagnosis of MS to be made, neurologists must be certain that two or more areas of the central nervous system are involved. These will be visible as lesions on MRI scans. This is because other central nervous diseases share some of the same warning signs, and some MS-type symptoms can have quite another cause. Symptoms must either be visible during a minimum of two distinct relapses separated by an interval of several months in relapsing-remitting MS, or as persistent deterioration over several months in primary progressive MS, for a certain diagnosis to be made.

Unpredictability and fluctuation are characteristic of MS symptoms. You never know when they are going to appear or disappear, how long they will stay and how intensely they will be experienced. Symptoms are at their most troublesome during relapse – that is when they appear, intensify and generally make their presence felt. During remission they generally ease up, and rarely persist as strongly – often they can clear away completely. Certain symptoms hang on with grim determination, but most are transient.

Symptoms come in varying strengths. The majority are only felt in a mild way, so you may even begin to believe you are imagining them. But just as you are getting used to a certain symptom it may vanish like a will-of-the-wisp, and it's only then, without it around, that you are convinced that it was for real. It's amazing how much one can put up with that's not normal; no wonder people with MS feel relief and an exhilarating feeling of well-being when a symptom goes away. Sometimes you read about a symptom, or hear talk of one, and are surprised to discover that what had always been shrugged off as a passing inconvenience actually merits the term 'symptom'. However, it is also an inescapable fact that for a few people MS symptoms can be severe, devastating and at times extremely persistent. In such circumstances it seems as if they will never ease off. Sadly, in a very small percentage of cases that is true, but normally there is some let-up. Symptoms that persist indefinitely can be really dispiriting unless some way is found of incorporating them into life rather than constantly fretting to be rid of them.

In the light of what you have just read you may well be anxious and frightened about the symptoms that can result from demyelination – quite understandably – and it is not surprising if people with MS find themselves shying away from meeting other people who are disabled with MS; they fear that the symptoms they see may afflict them in turn. What they overlook is the fact that MS is renowned for its fluctuating range of symptoms, varying in intensity and duration. Sitting in a wheelchair in the morning doesn't inevitably mean you still need to be in one in the afternoon.

Another understandable fear arises from the fact that symptoms appear and disappear as if at will. If you are currently troubled by a particular symptom, the possibility that it will just go gives hope. The reverse, when you are in remission and symptom-free, is more threatening. This is a threat that will not go away, a 'sword of Damocles', and only the person experiencing this fear can choose whether to ignore it and get on with living, or else spend time agonizing over what could happen. Giving way to negative thinking does not help. Being positive and realistic does. It is important to keep in mind that the body is made to revert to healthy balance and fullest function. The positive set of the mind will be a vital factor in this taking place. It is also true that the central nervous system, in particular, has amazing powers of healing. There is evidence, too, that myelin can be repaired. *Remyelination* is possible in the peripheral nerves, and nerve fibres can grow again. There is in fact the very real potential for MS symptoms to disappear permanently.

The next section of this chapter includes a comprehensive list of symptoms. You may be relieved to find your troublesome symptom isn't unique to you but within the range of MS normality. Remember again that some symptoms can be caused by something other than MS.

Everyone is different in the way they cope with their symptoms. A few capitalize on very little, and take great pleasure in sharing what they have been through, often exaggerating it. It serves to get them an audience for a short time, and they feel better for having dumped the load. Others, different in personality, accept the need to talk through what it feels like having to put up with symptoms. By talking about their experience to the sort of people who will offer understanding and support, and by releasing some of the associated tensions, emotions and fears, they are able to cope.

Symptoms
The invisible symptoms

These are the symptoms the person with MS is acutely aware of and discomforted by. They are the ones the non-MS person cannot see, never dreams exist, ignores or belittles, and for which only grudging sympathy is given. Sometimes they are the most troublesome of the lot. Their onset can be very rapid.

Peculiar sensations.   The most bizarre symptoms defy imagination and description. How can you explain the irritation of a trickling, twitchy feeling down a leg, hot and sweaty – or cold and clammy – feet or hands, the unrelieved heaviness of limbs? Most people have experienced pins and needles, but rarely for days at a time. Then there is a creeping numbness, that often starts in the feet and works its way gradually to the waist.

Impairment of touch results in a multitude of tingling sensations, many of which can be painful. Walking can be experienced as floating, trudging through water or snow, or making your way over eggs. Your whole body image can be disturbed, as if you don't know where different parts of the body are. The head feels detached from the body, and sight feels limited to a thin slit of vision.

Sensitivity to heat is a symptom that can commonly cause a temporary worsening of other MS symptoms.

Fatigue.   To relatives and close friends, fatigue can seem like a convenient symptom. It is the sort of symptom you might use to escape work if you didn't have MS and weren't the sort of person who habitually saw a task through to the bitter end. Sometimes fatigue is a permanent symptom that drags around with you. At other times it creeps up unnoticed, and when it becomes apparent, it's too late. The typical pattern is to start on a project – cleaning, walking, dancing, whatever – and perform quite normally until suddenly energy goes and you seize up or flop. The energy loss can be so immediate that you are taken quite by surprise. It is freqently accompanied by a dazed feeling and inability to communicate through excessive weakness. The fatigued person with MS is unable to enter into arguments or work out reasons. There is a partial shutdown and all incentive to communicate goes. Very occasionally people fall into slumber. Everything becomes too much of an effort, even thinking. Naturally, unless this symptom is understood and

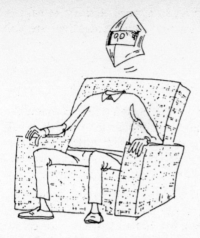

. THE HEAD FEELS DETACHED FROM THE BODY AND
SIGHT FEELS LIMITED TO A VISOR OF VISION...

accepted it has very adverse effects on relationships. More will be said about fatigue in Chapter 4.

Vertigo/dizziness.   One of the disturbing symptoms of MS some people experience is vertigo. It can vary from a little light-headed dizziness to feeling the world is turning upside down and tipping you off it. It can also be accompanied by nausea, vomiting, and an inability to walk straight – or at all.

Bladder problems.   The pressing need to pass water frequently and urgently is a distressingly unwelcome symptom. It limits your excursions to ones where a loo is in quick reach. Although it's no joking matter, it does help if you can deal with it in a light-hearted manner. On a theatre visit, Barbara was confronted with a long queue outside the ladies' loos. In desperation she shouted out that she had MS and had to get to the toilet immediately. At once doors flew open and she was able to take her pick. A bold exclamation that brought instant response and a few chuckles!

Sometimes the reverse is the problem and urine is retained, causing uncomfortable feelings of being bloated. This is most often a problem for women rather than men.

Incontinence.   This is a symptom dreaded by people with MS. Like other MS symptoms it can come without warning and disappear again like magic. It may be partial or total, and affect the bladder and/or bowels. Constipation may or may not accompany it.

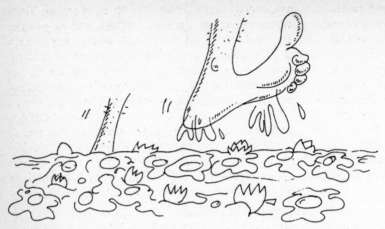

WALKING CAN BE EXPERIENCED AS FLOATING, TRUDGING
THROUGH WATER OR MAKING YOUR WAY OVER EGGS...

Pain.   Many persons with MS stress that they suffer a fair amount of pain of various types. It is only recently that some in the medical profession have been forced to admit the reality of pain in MS. Many different types of pain can be experienced: numb aching; pins and needles; tingling sensations; sharp shooting and stabbing pains; dull, gnawing nerve pains in an arm or leg; aching eyes like in a bad toothache; backache due to the strain of walking with difficulty; muscle spasms and cramps, with legs shooting out straight or bending sharply – most often in bed at night. The head and face can also be affected, and *trigeminal neuralgia* is sometimes experienced. This is an agonizing nerve pain in one side of the face; it lasts only a few seconds, and is accompanied by an involuntary contortion of the facial muscles that looks like a grimace.

Hearing.   Although deafness and tinnitus resulting from a brain-stem plaque are rare, some MS sufferers report impairment of their hearing. It is not so much that one cannot hear the sounds as that they don't seem to 'unscramble' sufficiently to make complete sense.

The inner ear is responsible for balance, and there is evidence in MS of loss of position-sense and the resulting problems of loss of balance.

Sight.   Sight is being included under the heading of invisible symptoms because many visual difficulties are usually transitory and rarely stay long enough to be noticeable to an observer. They are, however, symptoms that can distress, frighten and aggravate. No one likes having problems with their sight. Many people with MS report blurred or double vision (*diplopia*) or vision with blind spots (*scotomata*) as an early symptom of MS which normally clears up. There may also be temporary spells when there is a dimming of colour appreciation, and times when contrasts of shade are not as sharp as normal. Fifteen per cent of persons with MS experience *optic* or *retrobulbar neuritis*. *Nystagmus* is another problem and is when rapid eye movements are made, especially when looking from side to side. There can also be problems with moving both eyes together. A few people will experience permanent total or partial loss of sight, with a severe loss of central vision.

Sexual problems. These will be dealt with in detail later, but it is important to include them here since they can have a serious effect on relationships and cause considerable distress. Men with MS may find themselves unable to sustain an erection long enough for satisfactory intercourse. Women may experience an absence of vaginal sensation, or a distortion of it. Both men and woman may suffer from diminished arousal.

Emotions. With so much going on in the body and so many readjustments needing to be made, it is inevitable that people with MS are going to experience a wide range of emotions. There is also evidence that MS can cause magnified emotional reactions, with marked swings of mood as a consequence. Sometimes you cannot help but react with increased emotion, without any rhyme or reason. At other times, the emotional state may be accepted as appropriate – following initial diagnosis, for instance, or after a relapse or crisis.

Memory and concentration. At times you may recognize problems to do with memory loss, and find yourself waiting for the wrong bus or entering the wrong shop, for example. Your friends may take it lightly, but it can prove embarrassing and very inconvenient for you. You need to accept it is a symptom of MS, and be able to recognize it when it happens. In a similar way, you may become aware of marked problems with concentration or reasoning, problems which may interfere noticeably with the sort of work you do.

Psychological reactions. It is not uncommon to find yourself involved in a mental battle as you try to distinguish between the reality of what's going on in your body and what you fear you are imagining about yourself. Some people side-step the truth about how fatigued they actually are and what symptoms they are having to put up with. Instead, for various reasons, they interpret them in predominantly psychological terms. This usually means they blame themselves for what has gone wrong in their bodies. It doesn't help one whit, but it is their way of coping for the time being. It also has the effect of confusing family, friends and doctors as to what is really going on, and can thus make it harder for them to provide understanding and caring support.

The visible symptoms

These are the symptoms everyone can see. Obviously troublesome, they also attract attention. If you are confined to a wheelchair or walking with difficulty because of MS, you are noticed. You fit the classic picture of the disease, and people react to it. Whether they smother you with attention or studiously ignore you, they cannot help but register the reality that you have MS. There is no denying visible symptoms.

And yet, despite their appearance, they need not be any more troublesome than the invisible ones. Visible symptoms fluctuate too in their duration and intensity. What is here today may indeed be gone tomorrow, or the day after.

Weakness. This may be limited to weakness in part of the body, or it may be an overall feeling of not having your usual amount of strength. It shows as you drag a leg, find climbing stairs a problem, or walk instead of running. It shows when you sit down to iron or mend a plug. It shows whenever you flop into a chair or bed when you would normally have kept going. Others may not always immediately attribute it to MS, but they are clearly puzzled by this unaccustomed weakness.

To get rid of it, you may try all the common 'pick-you-ups', and follow advice to 'snap out of it' and 'pull yourself together'; but this is MS weakness, which is physiologically induced and can't be switched off at will.

Walking difficulties. For a while, you can cover up obvious stiffness as a result of over-exercise or a matter of age, but other walking problems aren't quite as easy to explain away. Lack of co-ordination, loss of balance, knees that give way so that you trip or topple over, the ataxic gait that resembles a drunken stagger – these are much more difficult to explain. Leg muscles can become weakened or paralysed. Feet (and hands too) can suffer from cramp-like contractions. Thus walking can be made difficult in many ways. Getting from one place to another becomes a strategic operation, and you resort to using sticks, frames, scooters or wheelchairs to make getting around easier and faster.

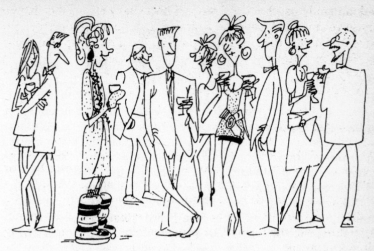

IT'S CERTAINLY NO FUN NEEDING TO WEAR BOOTS OR WOOLLEN SOCKS WITH PARTY GEAR...

Problems with making movements. Another symptom is lack of control and co-ordination over controlled movements. The smooth, controlled movement you normally make to carry out specific actions such as putting on make-up, lighting a match, or picking up a tool or piece of equipment, becomes a clumsy, inaccurate one. Others notice that you drop things and have more than your fair share of accidents. You may sometimes suffer from wobbly, shaking movements or tremors as you try to fulfil an everyday task. Muscle tone is altered and can produce spasticity or muscle stiffness which can affect movement. Messages just aren't getting through without interference, and it is showing in how you move.

Speech. If the tongue and other muscles involved in speaking are impaired, problems with speech may result. This may show in a minor way like the slowing down of speech, especially when you are tired. Often, speaking becomes slurred or jerky and garbled, like a mechanical toy. Naturally this can become a barrier to communication and cause distress to everyone involved in a conversation. This symptom is normally a later one.

The effects of poor circulation. These can become visible if your limbs – notably your feet – become very cold as a result, and you need to wear something warm. It's certainly no fun needing to wear boots or woollen socks with party gear. Ankles very often swell up, and you can feel quite uncomfortable.

Coping

Coping with a fluctuating disease like MS is a battle, and touches you at a deep psychological level. Whether MS affects you little by little, like fine rain that soaks you to the skin in time, or whether it grasps you in an iron grip, you cannot escape the fact that you now have to make space in your life for a chronic illness. You can try to squeeze it out but it won't disappear, except in natural remission. On the other hand, you can cope with it provided you dare to face up to what impact it will have on you – and move on, incorporating a new dimension in your life. Perhaps it is like the dark backcloth against which many shades of colour really stand out. While no one can welcome having MS, it can be turned to advantage. It needn't be a disaster, and you can still like living with MS! I am always struck by the countless times I've heard young people with MS confess that once they have got over the initial shock of learning to live with MS, they realize their diagnosis has given them an opportunity to take stock. Hesitantly, for they do not see themselves as heroic, they express a grudging gratitude that something like MS has pushed them to re-evaluate their lives. How, and what psychological barriers need confronting, are matters dealt with later in the book.

2

MS diagnosis and its consequences

Diagnosis

Diagnosis is a pivotal point. There was life before MS, life continues after it and the diagnosis stands starkly between. There is no one with MS who does not remain acutely aware for a long, long time, if not forever, of when, where, how and by whom his or her diagnosis was or was not made clear. MS diagnosis is a loaded term, and in an uncanny way never fails to arouse a gamut of strong feelings and reactions.

Is there a right time to make a diagnosis of MS? It is devastating to be given it too soon, and infuriating to be held out on. It would take more than the wisdom of Solomon to judge the time that was right for everyone. But by far the majority would prefer a clear diagnosis sooner rather than later. If your doctor decides to hold on to his suspicions and wait until there is no shadow of doubt clinically and from objective tests, you may well find you are so unwell or even disabled that his approach appears to ignore the obvious. (Quite a proportion of people with MS have guessed their diagnosis first.) If you are not yourself suspicious and prone to self-diagnosis, there is no doubt that your family and friends will have bombarded you with a thousand and one reasons for your condition.

It has been estimated that approximately three-quarters of the people with MS are told their diagnosis by a doctor. The rest discover the truth from a relative or by other means.

Making the diagnosis

There is no specific test for diagnosing MS. The sclerosis, plaques or lesions responsible for the damage cannot be seen with the naked eye. They can, however, be located in various ways. Often medical history together with physical examination provide sufficient information for a firm diagnosis. Other objective laboratory tests are sometimes required as confirmation. When attempting to confirm whether or not someone is suffering from MS, doctors will be listening for many different types of information. They will want to know when and at what age any of the symptoms became noticeable. They will be interested in where in the body symptoms have occurred, what sensations they have caused, and what effects they have had. They will need to be satisfied that a minimum of two separate areas of the central nervous system have been involved. One of two patterns with regard to time should become obvious: either at least two clear-cut episodes of interference because of demyelination, each lasting a reasonable period of time and separated from each other by a time gap, or the slow progressive development of one pattern of symptoms over a long period of time. A pattern of relapse and remission may also point to a diagnosis of MS.

The patient's medical history is usually corroborated by the findings of a physical examination by a neurologist. Part of this examination of the central nervous system will involve testing reflex pathways; for example, by tapping the knee with a surgical hammer. Measuring how much sensation there is in response to a stimulus is done by the pin-prick and/or cotton-wool test. In addition to reflexes and sensations, checks will be made on co-ordination, walking, standing, grip, eye movements and the functioning of the optic nerve. With MS the doctor will normally find some objective abnormality. In these ways he begins to build up a picture of which nerve pathways are currently affected. Illnesses other than MS must be positively eliminated first.

It must be stressed that an MS diagnosis is always a clinical one based on definite criteria. It isn't a diagnosis snatched out of the air when all other likely diseases have been ruled out. Your doctor must be satisfied that your symptoms and findings cannot be explained by anything other than MS.

Tests to aid diagnosis

When a diagnosis of MS is strongly suspected but has not been proven by physical examination and clinical evaluation of your case history, laboratory tests can be used. The most common tests include:

Evoked potential.   As demyelination has the effect of slowing down the rate at which messages are transmitted along the nerve pathways, *evoked potential* tests are often given. These measure how fast the central nervous system can respond to rapidly repeated stimuli.

The most common of these tests is the *visual evoked response* (VER). You sit in front of a screen with an alternating chequer-board pattern. Electrodes, lightly glued onto your scalp, record how quickly the brain responds to what the eyes see and a computer print-out records the information. It takes half an hour to have this test and it causes no discomfort at all.

Two other tests that operate along similar lines are one to test hearing ability – *brainstem auditory* testing (BAEP) and another to assess the sensory reaction of the body to touch – *somatosensory* testing (SEP).

Scanners.   The central nervous system can be scanned by the widely available CAT scanner or the rarer *magnetic resonance imaging* (MRI) scanner.

The traditional CAT scanner uses X-rays to produce cross-sectional pictures of the brain. Sometimes a dye is injected into the central nervous system to show up the sclerosis more clearly. As scar tissue is usually only visible during relapses, this test must be administered during an exacerbation to give any proof of demyelination. There is no discomfort involved in having a scan, and a very minimal risk from X-ray exposure or possible allergic reaction to the dye.

The MRI is a far superior and more sophisticated scanner. It has a remarkable sensitivity, picking out the smallest plaques, including those 'silent' ones not associated with any reported symptom. Its images or pictures are created without using X-rays. It is a computer-assisted imaging technique in which you are exposed to a strong magnetic field. As the sclerosis can be measured and viewed three-dimensionally with the MRI, it is now possible to obtain detailed information of what exactly is happening to the plaques, and to be precise about any changes and new damage. This scanner can be of enormous help in diagnosis, provided it is used in conjunction with clinical information. Its greatest potential, however, is its use, still in the early stages, in assessing the effects of treatment.

Lumbar puncture.   A *lumbar puncture* can give results which confirm an MS diagnosis. In this test a small amount of *cerebrospinal fluid* (CFS) is extracted for laboratory analysis. What this fluid contains in 90 per cent of persons with MS is antibodies, evidence of inflammation in the central nervous system. (Specifically, increased levels of gamma globulin and oligoclonal bands are being looked for.) In the early stages of MS it is rare for positive findings to show up.

Lumbar punctures are given less often today. They can cause some discomfort, and some people suffer from bad headaches afterwards.

It is best to remain lying down immediately after and if a

headache develops. If you do get any unpleasant side-effects, resting horizontally for as long as you need to is the best antidote.

Electromyography.   This is a technique used to measure how long it takes a nerve impulse to travel along the central nervous system to a muscle. It involves using an electromagnet together with electrical stimulation of the spinal cord.

Ways in which the diagnosis is made

Helpfully.   The open and frank telling of an MS diagnosis by a trusted GP or neurologist works well if there is already a caring relationship. It takes time for the implications to sink in, and a future appointment will need to be made for the patient (and partner, or parents) to come back and ask all those questions that shoot right out of your mind at times of stress, shock and an overload of new information. Sometimes doctors will involve a third party (such as a social worker), when they give the diagnosis so that there is another contact in a newly-forming health team which will operate to give support in the future as needed. A social worker can make more time available to discuss exactly what the doctor said and what effect it will have on general lifestyle. He or she can point out other sources of information and support, such as the local branch of the MS society or a group for the newly-diagnosed. Whether you have the disease or live close to someone who has you may want to know a lot more about MS and what you can expect. It is appropriate for your doctor and his team to offer you that support, and to give the facts realistically and with optimism.

You are likely to have some very real fears. These need to be aired and faced, not dismissed, and at the same time you need to take in very clearly the fact that no one can predict the outcome of your MS, nor be sure what repercussions there will be for you, your family or your friends.

Unhelpfully.   There is double pain when the diagnosis is given badly, in an off-hand and dismissive way by some medical official. 'Oh well, what can you expect when you've got MS?' is occasionally the first confirmation that you have the disease. There is no regard for your feelings or the shock you experience. It was most likely assumed that you already knew, and so the doctor was simply stating what was for him a medical fact of life. Rarely does the teller take a second look at you while he's spilling the beans, and so he misses the devastating effect his words have on you.

If this has been your experience, you know how destructive it can

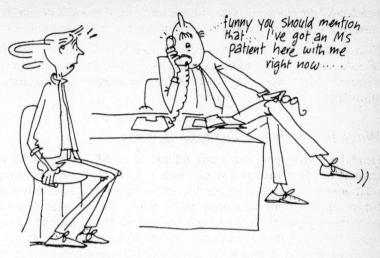

..THERE IS DOUBLE PAIN WHEN THE DIAGNOSIS IS GIVEN BADLY IN AN OFF-HAND DISMISSIVE WAY...

be. It need not be stressed that however busy medical professionals are, meticulous care must be taken to avoid this way of giving a diagnosis. Even if it was a genuine mistake, it ranks as a blunder, and you have every right to feel upset. It is as if you don't matter as a person with feelings. What is worse, you are generally denied the opportunity to discuss the implications of your diagnosis. Because it is assumed you already know and because you are probably too shocked to say anything much, the natural time to talk about what MS is, and how you are likely to be affected, passes without useful comment on either side.

To someone else. Fortunately it happens less frequently nowadays that a diagnosis is shared first with a partner or parent(s). Sometimes a relative can keep such information secret for many years before it is eventually revealed. When it is, the relationship with that person is likely to take a knocking. Sometimes it deteriorates badly, and distrust remains for ever between the two. Someone with MS may feel resentment at the withholding of information that was rightfully theirs all along. On the other hand, relatives have had an additional burden of secrecy and anxiety to cope with, on top of their own personal reactions to the diagnosis.

Very few wish they had never been told and kept shielded from the truth. Those who do are unable or unwilling to cope with anything unpleasant in life that touches them. It isn't so much the

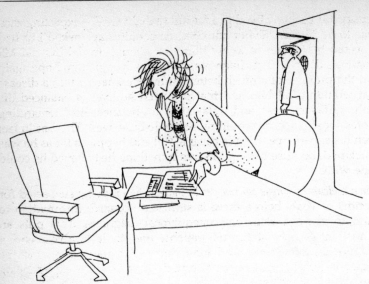

DEVIOUS DISCOVERY - YOU MAY HAVE DISCOVERED YOUR DIAGNOSIS
BY READING YOUR MEDICAL NOTES UPSIDE DOWN WHILE THE
DOCTOR WAS OUT...

facts of MS that they struggle with as the facts of life and their own personalities.

Devious discovery. If you have MS, you may have discovered your diagnosis by steaming open a letter, getting hold of your medical notes left lying about, or reading them upside down while the doctor was out of the room.

If so, you needed to know and were ready to be told. It may be that some doctors sense this and test out their patients' readiness by allowing notes to be easily available. This smacks of encouraging deviousness.

If you have a certain or even probable diagnosis, you have the right to be told how certain or uncertain it is. Keeping back such information leads to much anger and resentment. It is a fundamentally patronizing attitude that destroys a good patient-doctor relationship. It actually leaves you with the upper hand, not the doctor. You have to confront the doctor with your deviously gained information, or play dumb and wait for the revelation.

Assuming worse than the worst. Not being told a diagnosis directly can lead to more anxiety than is necessary. Frank was suddenly refused long-term insurance, and his cover was limited to one year. A highly intelligent man with many years of first-aid experience, he assumed he must be suffering from something far worse than MS.

For several years he lived in a fearful twilight world, expecting each year to be his last. Frank admitted he should have asked but had expected his doctor to know him well enough to tell him an MS diagnosis directly. The diagnosis of MS finally gave him hope again and the promise of a much better future. He knew it was a disease that wouldn't kill him and that provided he lived a balanced life with sufficient rest and relaxation to balance his demanding professional work, he would probably do quite well. This has in fact been his experience. His life became full and happy as far as he was concerned, because having MS was something he believed he could cope with.

When a clear diagnosis cannot yet be made.   MS may be suspected for months or years before there is sufficient objective information to hand to make a clear and unequivocal diagnosis. This puts an almost intolerable strain on patients and their families, and a distance between them and their doctors. It may seem as if the doctor is holding out on you, especially if you are experiencing inexplicable symptoms.

There is a very real dilemma for a doctor when MS is suspected but the right combination of clinical information and test results is not present. A patient wants to know why his or her body isn't functioning properly and so does the doctor, who needs to rule out diseases or conditions that may be more serious or treatable.

One common pitfall with neurological symptoms is the fact that those suffering from them tend to become introspective. Their symptoms are frightening, and even small ones take on a great significance. Because symptoms come and go and are bizarre in character, they sound neurotic. It's very easy for some persons with MS to sound hysterical and for doctors to take more notice of that than the suspected underlying organic problem. It follows that a doctor with such a patient may fear an increased hysterical reaction if he gives too early a diagnosis of MS which can't be cured or systematically controlled. More often than not, though, such a patient copes quite adequately with a definite diagnosis.

Not knowing the cause of symptoms is more frustrating; the greatest fear is always that of the unknown. You may imagine that valuable time is being lost, time that should be spent on treating your disorder. On diagnosis, your anxiety ceases to be hysterical, and assumes a natural level.

When a doctor cannot make a definite MS diagnosis with professional confidence, he will best give support by assuring a patient that he has heard and accepted all the evidence given. Sometimes you have to ask your doctor to do just that. It is vital that you know you are believed and can come back again and again to discuss the matter. If your doctor can honestly admit his reason for being unable (but not unwilling) to diagnose, your relationship is one to be trusted and highly valued.

What to do with an MS diagnosis

What you decide to do with the new information of an MS diagnosis will depend on your personality and how much of a trauma the diagnosis is. You may need to keep the diagnosis quiet. You need space and time to absorb and react to it in private or with a chosen few. You may even be determined not to reveal it to anyone. Perhaps you fear dismissal from work, being walked out on by your partner, being seen as a failure or even in some way responsible for your body malfunctioning.

On the other hand, you may have to broadcast the information so that other people will know immediately what is wrong. Perhaps you need others to understand what you have had to put up with. You need the truth to be out in the open. It may be just too much for one person to hold on to alone.

Between these two reactions there is a workable balance. Sharing the diagnosis invites support and caring. It gives a legitimate reason for making changes in lifestyle and redirecting energy and resources most efficiently. You are responsible for your own life, and can choose how you will relate to those in your world. You can do this well when you know how to cope with the inevitable consequences of an MS diagnosis.

Putting the past into perspective

Diagnosis is a point in life when you can dare to admit the full, uncomfortable reality of what is now an officially-confirmed part of yourself. The experience of the past begins to make sense now that there is this new information. It is a time to begin to unravel the mysteries of aggravating symptoms. It can be liberating to be able to name MS as the cause of a multitude of previously isolated and unrelated incidents. A diagnosis can have the effect of clearing confusion and lifting burdens that have made life puzzling and difficult, and have soured relationships as a consequence.

A firm diagnosis allows you time for self-justification – the experience prior to diagnosis was real, and had not been simply imagined. It also buys you a breathing space; time is needed to absorb the fact that MS is part of your life ahead. In a sense, it moved in permanently long ago and its demand for accommodation is being heard loud and clear only now.

For most people there follows a time of facing up to the facts and the challenge of daring to start again. The reality of MS is that you may not have enough energy to cope both with physical symptoms and with the essential process of re-evaluation at the same time. However, it is helpful to tie up loose ends from the past and then be free to focus attention on what you need to cope with here and now. This will involve looking at many aspects of life that you have previously pushed into a corner and ignored. There is always a danger that those closest will not want stones from the past to be turned over. They may not see any necessity for change, and will cling on to preserving the *status quo* – or alternatively, make a quick exit.

In a sense, every MS diagnosis is a shock. Even if it has been suspected for a long time and comes as a relief from the uncertainty of no diagnosis, it is still a shock. It is a shock that numbs and is unreal. It is a shock that enrages and is unfair. It is a shock that can hurl you into panic and despair. It is also an inescapable shock, and one normal reaction to such shock is to attempt to ignore its repercussions.

The discovery of new, strong and powerful feelings is as painful and confusing as discovering you have MS. Feelings make themselves felt sooner or later. They exist, like toes or fingers, as a natural part of you. At diagnosis you and those close to you may not know quite what you are feeling. Your feelings may seem to be out of control or getting in the way of your thinking. You may not be sure why you are reacting so strongly, nor clear what the reaction is about. Your body cannot escape the reality of feelings and their effect on it. Unhappiness or pleasure, depression or exhilaration have a consequent reaction in the body, an 'emotional tone' that cannot be ignored. Add this additional overlay to MS symptoms and diagnosis, and it's understandable that there is a confused welter of feelings and a struggle over who you are as a person right now.

In this situation the focus needs to be on finding your identity afresh. At diagnosis you take a knocking. It is almost as if you step out of your skin, without a new one to step into. The only way of coping with it is to focus on the reality of what you feel, the way you are behaving and what symptoms you are experiencing.

It is a fact much overlooked that everyone grows up expecting to live a full life with a normally healthy body. Of all else in life this is the most common expectation of stability: you seem programmed to expect health to be more stable than anything or anyone else. That is why so many elderly people are distressed by the inevitable problems of getting old. Old people have a resistance to regarding the slowing down and gradual deterioration that come with old age as normal or natural, whereas these things seem perfectly understandable in an old person if you are still young. Similarly, if you are not disabled it is merely a matter of course that a disease like MS will have some disabling effect.

So what feelings do people experience when it seems their right to normal health has been denied and they are forced to accept a diagnosis of MS? It is perfectly normal to feel sorrow and loss, anger and frustration, fear and isolation, together with conflicting feelings of total denial followed by resignation and acceptance. Each of these feelings needs to be understood, worked through and adjusted to if you are to function smoothly again.

Feelings of sadness and loss

No loss in life can be ignored. The natural reaction to loss is to express your sorrow. It can be called mourning or grieving, and is part of bereavement. Although there are some things in life people are glad to lose, you always struggle, kick and fight when whatever you value is torn from you, as if part of you is torn away with it.

What is it you perceive you have lost when newly diagnosed with MS? It may be any or all of the following. You lose a normally active body and gain a body suffering from a named disease, MS. You lose a body that you have always believed functioned at your command and gained a body that clearly functions in its own sweet way. You lose a body that is averagely active and on the go, for a body that is fatigued. You may lose – at least temporarily – legs that hop, skip, and jump, for ones that drag, limp and stumble. You may lose arms and legs that put on make-up or work a lathe; eyes that locate the oncoming traffic without having to turn your head; speech that is lucid and flowing; a brain that remembers in a flash and deals efficiently with impressions and situations. You may lose a lifestyle in which you are always in control, doing what you want, when you want, without restrictions from inside yourself, because suddenly with MS you aren't functioning properly. Each of these losses may result in obvious spin-offs – loss of self-confidence, and even loss of work, social life, family and friends. This is how it can be when feelings of sadness in response to loss sweep over you. Your appetite may go, your sleep may be interrupted, you may feel depressed and despondent. What you need is to find a way to start being put together again.

There are three steps to deal with sadness:

- Accept your sadness as a normal and healthy reaction to the loss or losses you perceive after diagnosis.
- Find ways of expressing the sadness so that it comes out into the open. Holding in sad feelings is an immense effort, and consumes the energy you need to fight MS.

- If you can trust someone to be with you when you need to talk about your losses and sorrow, it will help you to release the feelings in the most healing way. Some people find through psychotherapy that the presence of an understanding person and, if appropriate, a reassuring touch when one cries have a deep and healing effect.

Facing loss at diagnosis

Any interference with your normal lifestyle as a result of having MS results in a feeling of loss. Loss of health is never easy to come to terms with, and cannot be ignored. If you want to go on living meaningfully, you have to adjust to it. After an MS diagnosis people will become aware of both physical and emotional changes and of changes in the way they relate to other people, and some of these will feel like losses.

It is possible to move through this time of loss and learn to adjust. It's rather like a bereavement, and involves going through various stages that take you from confusion about MS to integration of it in your life. The initial reaction to loss is to deny it and refuse to believe it. You cannot believe it's actually happening to you and is really true. It may mean not wanting to hear about MS or meet anyone else with MS. You do all you can to prove to yourself and the world at large that you could not possibly have MS.

Then comes the resistant period when you may be very energetic, avidly seeking advice and investigating possible cures and treatments. Inside, you admit your MS is real, but find it hard to accept its impact. You need to find ways of beating the disease. Your energy may come across in a belligerent way, and other people may find you angry. Doctors often bear the brunt of angry outbursts, for this is the stage when those newly-diagnosed feel they have a right to know about their illness, and their doctor may not have all the answers.

Once the reality of an MS diagnosis is faced, however reluctantly, a person begins to feel in control of life again, learning how to cope with emotions and feelings, even if the feelings are negative ones, and recognizing what it is like to feel isolated emotionally too. It is a bargaining stage in which the aim is to win the battle between accepting that what is left is good and letting go of what was and has gone. It takes determination to emphasize the positive, but it is a good way of overcoming depression. When you are willing to disclose that you have MS and what that means for you, you help others to respond more appropriately. It helps to reach out for support from others, whether they be individuals or groups that focus on coming to terms with MS. The sooner it is possible to accept any help that is on offer, and to adjust to having MS, the better the quality of life will be. What must be remembered with MS, however, is that this affirming process is often interrupted by exacerbations. Just as you feel you are able to cope, you suffer a setback, and as a result may find yourself back at the denial stage or resistant period. It is rather like a game of snakes and ladders.

The final stage of the bereavement process is when a person is able to accept MS and all it entails as simply part of life. By now it is possible to subordinate some of the needs a person with MS has, in order to fit in with the requirements of others. MS is no longer the total preoccupation, but can be integrated into everyday life. It is no longer something to be ashamed of and people find they can ask for and receive the help and support they need.

Going through the process of bereavement is one that not only people with MS but also their family and friends need to experience. What is special about adjusting to MS is that you may have to do it more than once. It lasts well until the next relapse or exacerbation comes along. Then the process begins all over again. Despite that, if you have once adjusted well to MS, you will be able to do it again, working through the stages even if they are slow and painful, because you already know the relief that comes at the end.

What happens if you *don't* mourn your loss, or get stuck at one of the stages, is that your life is less rich and satisfying. On top of

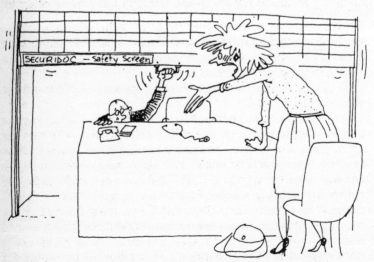

... DOCTORS OFTEN HAVE TO BEAR THE BRUNT OF ANGRY OUTBURSTS ...

having MS, you may feel depressed. You may lose sleep and appetite. Feelings of despondency will increase, and this will lead to your feeling less than positive about yourself. If it continues, you'll start to see yourself in a different – and negative – light, and will push to one side formerly valued plans and goals for the future. There will be a negative effect on your relationships too, for with depression come feelings of rejection by others and an increasing sense of isolation. Instead of growing to maturity, your personality will stagnate and you will find yourself taking on the stereotyped behaviour of a depressed person who believes that MS is the end of the road.

Only by facing up to the losses that are an inevitable part of your MS and mourning them properly, can you avoid a spiral down into depression and be able to move upwards instead.

Feelings of anger and frustration

Anger is a natural reaction when something you want to do is not possible. Blocked goals result in frustration. MS may stop many of your goals from being realized. When you cannot do things because you or your partner's MS decrees no, angry feelings are bound to arise.

What do you do with this anger? Where should it be directed? How should it be released? The two natural reactions to anger are either to fight back or run away. Not acknowledging you are angry and holding on to it is unnatural and unhelpful. It may be better to:

- Accept anger as a normal and healthy reaction.
- Own your anger, and take responsibility for handling it in such a way that it does not harm you or anyone else. It can become a source of creative energy.
- Find safe and, if possible, productive ways of expressing these strong feelings. You may need to seek professional help from someone trained in psychotherapy to get started. If you have the physical energy, you may find that an activity like polishing the car, digging the garden, kneading dough or some other vigorous exercise is an excellent release of anger and frustration. If you are low in energy, you will not believe you could gain any benefit from using up that last ounce of 'go' on bothering to express your frustration. However, if you have the courage or are desperate enough to give it a go, you will find that a roar of frustration or a defiant shake of the fist will result in a physiological release of tension that is followed by a doubled resurgence of energy.
- Don't throw your anger at someone else and try to get him or

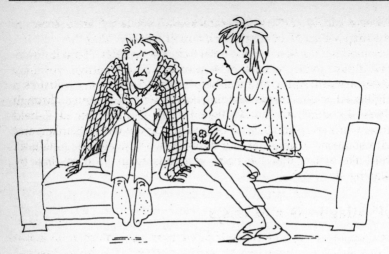

. CURLING UP SMALL , A BLANKET WRAPPED ROUND TIGHTLY,
AND WITH SOMEONE CARING THERE AS SUPPORT, WORKS WELL

her to take the blame. Again, own your feelings of anger, and your right to feel that way when what you want is denied. MS adds to life's frustrations but doesn't give you the right to lash out at family, friends and doctors when you feel angry.

- If there is something you can do to change and improve the situation, then work first of all on dealing healthily with the angry feelings. When they are released, you will have energy and a clearer mind to think of what options are open and the best way of going round the blocked goal.

The threat of fear

Fear can have a paralysing effect, or accelerate you into panic. An MS diagnosis is a fearful one. As it is a disease with fluctuating symptoms and a variable course, no one can be certain what will happen. It is normal to be fearful in the face of the unknown. Faith, and the support of loving people, can help contain the fear. So too can allowing yourself to be brave enough to look at what threat you are actually facing.

Talking through what would be the worst that could happen, and asking yourself what you would do then, very often results in the unexpected discovery that although unwelcome, the threat can be coped with. It won't remove the threat, but it will make it clear, and will release energy to cope with finding alternatives if they exist.

Better a single devil you've tracked to its lair than a score of imaginary goblins in every dark corner.

Sometimes you can't voice what your fear is, or can't pin it down. If you have someone close who wants to be supportive, you may like to try asking for physical help in the following way. Just as a frightened child needs holding close and reassuring through physical contact, so the frightened adult is strengthened if held close. Curling up small, wrapped round tightly with a blanket, and with someone caring there for support, works well. It is a natural, child-like action that the body responds to in its own time by relaxing slowly.

MS diagnosis and crisis

At diagnosis you find yourself faced with new information about yourself. It forces you to take stock, consider new challenges and discover strategies to help you cope. You could say it is a time of crisis. For a time after diagnosis, you and those close to you are caught up in a unique situation. Temporarily you may feel as if you are encapsulated in a bubble, isolated, cut off from the mainstream, halted, until you have had sufficient opportunity to reassess where you are, who you are and what direction you wish to go in. Every MS diagnosis produces shock waves whose ripples wash into every aspect of your life, and on to affect the lives of others you come in contact with, however fleetingly. Until the ripples have calmed down, the crisis continues.

What you experience at diagnosis may be your only crisis time with MS – or you may find other crises will follow. Much depends on the sort of person you are and the way you normally deal with unexpected situations. It makes a world of difference if you are able to face the crisis and discover ways of coping with MS that work for you. If you leave the crisis of diagnosis unresolved, it may mark the start of a long stage of conflict inside yourself.

What exactly is a crisis situation like? How do you know if you are going through a crisis? You first experience some signs of stress, and these can be physical or psychological or both. You tend to react in one of two ways: either you panic, or you feel like throwing the towel in. You feel overwhelmed, somewhat helpless and inadequate. It's not surprising then that you can't tackle life with your usual enthusiasm and efficiency. All you want is to get rid of the uncomfortable feeling of being knocked off balance, which is what crisis is about. It's too painful an experience for you to want to prolong it.

The other side of the shock of diagnosis is the positive relief it brings. On the one hand, it is so unexpected and so devastating; but on the other, you know now that you were right in your suspicions. On the one hand, it feels like the worst day of your life; on the other, it's better to know. On the one hand, you feel your whole world is tumbling in; but on the other, better the devil you know. For a time you may feel there's no point in going on; but once you've taken the diagnosis on board, you begin to feel that now you can get on and live again. At first you may just want to run away; but then you begin to accept that it's time to change and rebuild.

However you react, you register that having MS spells change. Nothing will be quite the same again. You will still be all you were before, positive and negative, but you will have a new and different perspective. This is the crux of the crisis around diagnosis. Even if it is a relief to have a name to label your health problem with, you still go through a time of crisis as you are forced to take stock.

If your MS is currently benign, you will still need to consider a fresh perspective on life. This may mean changing your priorities, accepting less ambitious goals, or at least being prepared to achieve them in a different way and with less pressure on time. Until you have made a reassessment of this sort, you are still in crisis.

Sometimes a diagnosis is revealed at a time when you are experiencing a considerable number of symptoms, a run of relapses, or increasing disability. Some symptoms have a direct effect on whether you can drive, work, socialize or continue to care for yourself independently. This is obviously a crisis situation too.

It is also a time of crisis for family and friends. They want to support you, and at the same time they have their own reactions and feelings to cope with. They experience the same range of emotions as the person with MS: anger about the unfairness and inconvenience of MS; sorrow over the pain and lost opportunities; fear of the unknown. On top of this, there is guilt because they don't have it and you do. Their relationship with you – and yours with them – will be affected as you each work through the crisis. They may try to 'make it better', or they may 'want out' at once. You need both time and a strategy to cope with crisis.

3

Living with MS

How to cope

The word 'cope' is often used as if it were a foolproof method of resolving any tricky situation. However, coping does not mean providing a ready-made solution to a problem. What it does mean is finding ways in which you can live with the problem and minimize its effects. Inevitably people cope with problems in a variety of ways. Although coping strategies are very much an individual matter, they can be approached in two ways: those of change and management.

Situations can be changed to suit your needs. By changing the situation, you remove your problem. This is a very good way of coping, for it ends in the problem being resolved. But not all problems and situations can be resolved; some are unchangeable. Unfortunately, this is true of MS. Despite its very changeable nature – in the sense that it comes and goes – MS is not going to go away. You cannot choose not to have it around any longer.

With something like MS, then, changing the situation is not a possible way of coping. As far as MS is concerned, the only changes you can make are not to the disease itself but in your reactions to it. So the situation doesn't change – your thoughts and feelings about it do. This is the management approach to coping. You may be unable to change the way your body behaves with MS, but you can learn to manage the way you react to it. This will not be a new skill to you, for all your life you have been managing your reactions to a host of situations. In this sense, MS is another new challenge for you to face, and you bring to it your previous coping skills – sharpened for most effective use.

Coping with work

MS has had such a bad press that the mere mention of its name conjures up, for some, pictures of rapidly accelerating paralysis. It is no wonder, then, that employers think twice before engaging someone with MS, and may try hard to ease out an existing employee who develops it. They need to know that paralysis is an exceptional symptom, and that most symptoms flare up and then either stabilize or die down again for a long period of time. Many people with MS can continue to cope with a perfectly normal working life, with little or no loss of working capacity. The effects of MS are in any case minimal for those with a mild form of the disease, and this is the norm. Even when an employee is visibly or more seriously affected, employers should also be encouraged to consider redeployment.

From time to time you will need to assess the effect of your MS on the work you do – whether outside or within the home setting. As soon as MS begins to interfere in any way with your ability to work, you need to begin to consider whether to introduce any changes that will make it practical for you to continue working.

It is difficult to know when to tell your employer about your MS. You will be reluctant, if not afraid, to do so because of the very real threat of being made redundant. It is perhaps understandable that if your MS interferes with your ability to do your work, your employer will consider taking some action. This can mean getting the sack but more often it involves squeezing you out by putting the pressure on you to 'choose' to go. It may mean redeployment, demotion, or simply no chance of promotion, all options you may feel are unfair. At best you may be offered a redundancy or settlement payment, and at worst thrown out of work on the pretext of legality; it is worth checking your legal rights.

If the symptoms you are currently experiencing are invisible, you may find it beneficial to explain that, though not obvious to anyone else, they are real. You should suggest new ways of tackling your job, or how conditions at work could be modified to make it easier for you to continue to work. If you hide behind invisible symptoms you are not only multiplying stress and strain for yourself as you try to minimize the effect, but also throwing yourself open to being misunderstood. Gloria managed to land a temporary clerical desk job some months after giving up her permanent teaching job. Its part-time hours and routine work suited her as she didn't need to leave her desk often. It soon became clear, though, that she too was expected to take her turn in fetching the drinks on a tray from the dispenser downstairs. She knew she'd have a problem managing the stairs and a full tray and made plausible excuses to avoid the task. Soon it blew up into a confrontation. The others clearly thought she was acting a bit above herself and to prove she wasn't, she went and got the drinks. When her boss found her struggling up the stairs, precariously balancing the drinks, he realized something else was perhaps to blame. Once the MS problem was made known, a compromise could be reached and good relations were restored.

Thus, invisible symptoms can prove more difficult to cope with than visible ones: urgency and frequency of incontinence become less of a problem if you can relocate near a toilet and your colleagues understand it's a common MS symptom. Fatigue that can sweep over you like a tidal wave so strong you have to rest for a while can be coped with if your employers agree to your taking rest periods and provide somewhere suitable for you to lie down. Working flexi-hours, taking work home to finish, or reducing to part-time employment may prove more suitable.

It may be possible in an office-type job to make up for work left incomplete due to fatigue or eyesight problems when you have got back your normal energy. But that approach will not work if you do manual work or just have to keep on the go – as in nursing, for instance. Heavy physical effort or intense mental strain day in and day out can cause a relapse or make symptoms worse. Sometimes it is possible to over-ride or mask symptoms by sheer determination, but this only works short-term. You find yourself getting through the week but collapsing exhausted at weekends, and getting through the day only to flop every evening. If work is a priority then you may accept this even if it's a steep price to pay. But the next day arrives before your energy reserves have been topped up sufficiently, and you run yourself into the ground. This is when you need to reassess how many hours per week you can work and whether you choose to carry on doing that type of work. Physical work involving exertion or fine, co-ordinated movements of hand, leg and eye may have to be given up and alternative work considered. This is what Nigel did. He was an optician in his late fifties when diagnosed with MS. Although he could no longer manage to work as an optician, he felt sure he could now make a pipe-dream a reality. At home he equipped a workshop with wood-turning equipment, and from a much-loved hobby grew a small but successful and rewarding business.

It is important not to become a limping liability at work. Falling over may be a safety hazard, especially if there is equipment around, and also dangerous for your own health. You may have to rethink your job so you can limit how much you move around. Using a scooter or wheelchair may become a safer, quicker way of getting around – perhaps even the only practical one. It will probably involve relocating to the ground floor or depending on a lift. Access to your place of work will have to be checked, and ramps, widened doorways, adapted toilets, and specified parking places provided. All employers are, in fact, encouraged to make full provision for disabled employees, but they often need pressurizing to do so. They would prefer the easier option of employing someone who is not disabled to having to cater for someone who is.

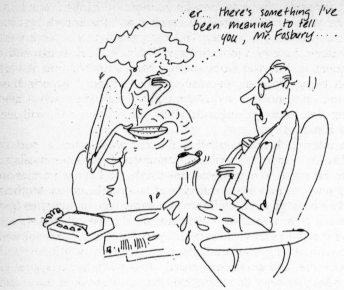

er... there's something I've been meaning to tell you, Mr. Fosbury....

IT'S DIFFICULT TO KNOW WHEN TO TELL YOUR EMPLOYER ABOUT MS

However, the fact that you can't rely on your walking may never interfere at all with your ability to perform your work well. If or when it becomes obvious to your workmates that you have a physical disability, they will be challenged to accept that this need not debar you from work. Mary has discovered that because she is excellent at her job, her colleagues completely ignore the fact that her scooter has become her legs. To compensate for her disability, she has chosen to focus on the quality of her work, and that's working well for her.

In general, employers and some colleagues manage very well when they know that the MS symptoms that cause problems at work include the obvious ones of not being able to get around at work, or travel to or from it easily. They deserve to be told how essential it is to be near a toilet sometimes. They also need information on MS fatigue and related problems such as poor concentration, memory lapses, slurring speech, and general low spirits and morale. Once they realize that all these symptoms normally fluctuate and disappear fast, they cope well enough.

Because loss of employment has such a devastating effect, you will do best to stay at work as long as you want to. Most people need to work for their own personal satisfaction as well as to remain financially independent. To be deprived of work is a blow that robs you of status, a regular routine, and the knowledge that you are contributing to society. This is especially true if you are the breadwinner. Loss of a job results in diminished self-worth and a subsequent withdrawal from society. Men with MS find it very difficult being workless, because society in general expects husbands to be the breadwinners. Also, without realizing it, wives tend to reject non-working husbands who, if they have MS, will feel doubly insecure.

It is relevant here to mention the chores that are a part of everyday life. Shopping, washing, cleaning and preparing meals all have to be done. Whether you are single, or have a partner or family, your MS may make this type of work difficult too. Mothers with MS who have young children at home to care for too often find housework is more than they can manage with the reduced energy and the symptoms they are experiencing. It is hard to ask for and get the type of help you want. Partners, relatives, neighbours and friends can be so supportive in practical ways. During a relapse or when disability persists, a mother may be forced to limit her running of the home to an organizing or co-ordinating role. The physical chores are undertaken by others, including home helps, but she uses her practised expertise to help plan and budget whenever possible. It is an option that allows her to make a valuable contribution, although it does have its share of frustrations – lacking, for example, the dubious pleasure of standing in long supermarket queues.

More and more people need to be better informed about the effects of MS on work. In Britain, government services, such as the Disablement Advisory Service, have been set up to address some of the problems involved. You can ask for medical advice from the Employment Medical Advisory Service (EMAS), and if you want to change your job, vocational assessment and guidance is available from the Employment Rehabilitation Centre (ERC) – for addresses see page 140. Disablement Rehabilitation officers (DROs) are available, through the local Job Centre, to help you to find work you can do.

Coping with pregnancy

You and your partner have the right to choose whether or not to have a child. It has to be your joint decision. Only you know how much you really want your own children. As responsible parents you will assess what this may mean, given the unpredictable course of MS. Bringing up children is rewarding and fun, but it is exhausting and demanding too. You need a lot of energy and

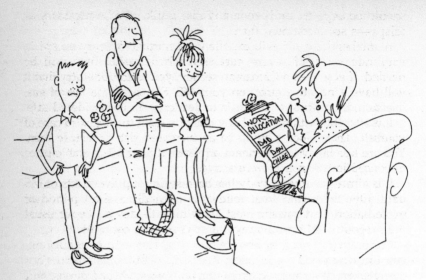

DURING A RELAPSE A MOTHER MAY BE FORCED TO
LIMIT HER RUNNING OF THE HOME TO AN ORGANISING OR
COORDINATING ROLE...

patience, and it helps to have sound finances. MS is not hereditary, but you need to appreciate that there is a genetic trait in MS that makes it ten times more likely than average that family members will develop it. The risk of a child of an MS parent developing MS itself is slight – one in a hundred – so most doctors would not consider the fact that a pregnant woman or her partner has MS as grounds for terminating the pregnancy.

Most women with MS seem to do well during pregnancy. Like women everywhere, some bloom and others feel rough when pregnant. Pregnancy won't protect you against all MS symptoms. Some of those you do experience could arise either from MS or from being pregnant. Many women report little change in the pattern of their MS during the first half of pregnancy but find improvement in the second half, with noticeably fewer exacerbations. This is probably to do with the way the body automatically functions to protect the unborn child.

It is wise to plan your pregnancy. If you can conceive while in remission, or wait until a couple of years after a severe relapse, you give yourself and your baby a good start. If you normally take drugs – such as those to control spasms or incontinence – it is best to come off them, following medical advice, before you get pregnant. Any long-term therapy of drugs or hyperbaric oxygen should be stopped before conception. During pregnancy, steroids should be avoided, and are in any case unlikely to be necessary as relapse is so uncommon then.

A mother with MS will experience a normal delivery except in very rare cases of severe paralysis, when special help will be needed. If you need a Caesarean section, you need not worry that it will have a negative effect on your MS. Similarly, the use of gas, injection or epidural anaesthesia to deaden pain is considered safe.

It is *after* the birth of your baby that you need to take extra care of yourself. There does seem to be an increased risk of relapse then. You are less likely to experience a relapse if your MS is stable prior to conception than if it were active.

It is almost as if your body has been storing up the effects of MS until after the birth. What follows is normally a short period of exacerbation, and you are most likely to settle down to your usual pre-pregnant MS condition within a year from conception.

Although you may not be able to stop a relapse from happening, you can do something to make it less likely and less severe. Find out what makes you tired and aggravates your MS symptoms, and avoid it. It is vital to get as much sleep and relaxation as you possibly can – you really can't get too much. Remember that breast-feeding can be very tiring for any mother, and causes some to feel anxious. It may be worth changing to an alternative way of feeding. All women benefit from practical help and understanding support as they adjust to motherhood. You deserve as much as you can get for the sake of your health, your baby and your family. This is the time to capitalize on the use of every labour-saving device and machine you can. Your priorities must be yourself and your baby, for it is your warm attachment that will give it the best start in life. Of course, you will sometimes feel insecure about being a mother. Most women do, and MS gives you an additional reason to feel that way. Mothers with MS often worry that their MS fatigue, exacerbations and relapses will stop them from being good mothers. In the end, your baby thrives because you are close and affectionate when you are with it, even for short spells. It is the relationship that really counts; baby really couldn't care less who does the housework, washing or cooking, so save your energy for your baby and get help with the rest. When you feel ready, it is important for your child's development that you include other loving people in his or her world, a safeguard if you can't be there. Children naturally have big, loving hearts, and respond to warmth and affection from other members of the family and friends. They deserve early on to have access to additional support and security when you may not be able to do a super-mum act.

No problem is too trivial to seek help for. Sometimes local mother and baby groups exist and can be an invaluable source of

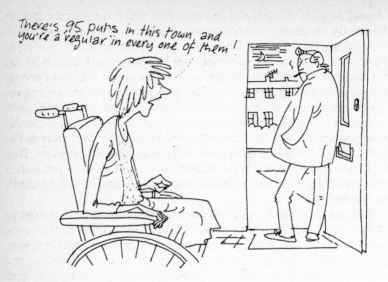

MS WILL INEVITABLY HIT THE MOST VULNERABLE SPOT IN A RELATIONSHIP...

reassurance and support. You need to know how much of what you are experiencing is the norm for *all* mothers; it's so easy to blame MS, and then to feel isolated and alone, with an additional burden to carry. And sharing what you are going through with your young baby will not only help you but support other mothers too.

Coping with your partner

MS threatens to have a negative effect on your relationship with your partner. There is plenty of evidence world-wide that divorce and separation are high in couples where one partner has MS. Any crisis such as MS will inevitably hit the most vulnerable spot, and this is most dramatically true in close relationships. In theory, the one person you can hope to be closest to, best understood by, cared for and loved by is your partner – and this may be your experience. But it could be that your relationship has never reached such intimacy and never will. You may be enjoying a secure, fulfilling relationship or putting up with one already cracking with stress and strain. MS is going to force the issue, if there is one.

It is too easy to blame MS for souring a relationship. MS is not to blame, but it can be a trigger. It puts your partnership under a glaring spotlight that picks out its existing weaknesses as well as its strengths. What counts is how well you and your partner got on before the diagnosis. If you skated along without ever needing to resolve any major issues, MS is one to get your teeth into. If all you have ever done is to confront problem after problem, MS can become just one more to work on, or one too many. MS can become the focus of a struggle you are already waging in which once again you try to resolve the inequalities in your relationship. Some use it to force a change in the other, so that their way of maintaining the relationship can win. This time the stakes are high, and there is the potential for far-reaching damage to be done to both partners. This is a good time to evaluate realistically what your relationship consists of, and to assess what each of you is willing to contribute to its success.

Both you and your partner must come to terms with the extent to which you are able to cope with MS. Your experience of it will be shared – but from a different perspective. You will both struggle with strong feelings – feelings that may be kept firmly under control, but may equally seep out or explode. You may find yourself wanting to lash out at your partner or keep a distance, to protect or reject, and often to manipulate. It takes courage to admit that with MS you both hurt. That is the way it was for Janet, who looked after her husband with devoted care and took over the role of breadwinner when in his later years he became severely disabled. David could never talk to her or anyone else about his MS. They coped, accepting the strain of never daring to say aloud what a hell of a disease MS had become. After his death Janet needed to share her hatred of what living with MS was like. She made particular mention of how normal he had looked from the waist up but how much notice she had taken of his hands which in his late sixties had become visibly twisted. She hated the memory of those hands; for her they symbolized the disability of MS. Physical disability and day-to-day nursing care get to partners. They suffer. They agonize when they give all they can, knowing it will never repair the disability. It is pointless trying to decide who gets the worst deal. Both of you do.

It is an indisputable fact that while you cannot escape your MS, your partner may want to – and decide to. Only a small minority walk out early on, without giving you and your MS a go. But we all differ in what we are prepared to put up with. It can happen that sickness and disability are the very things your partner most fears and really cannot cope with. Anything else would be alright, but not something like MS. Some have already been looking for an excuse to leave, and in MS find one they can justify. However, it can work the other way round too. Maria quickly made up her mind upon her diagnosis that although she was prepared to cope with having MS, she was not prepared to put up with her husband too. She immediately started divorce proceedings.

There are certain factors that help to cement a relationship and give it a sound enough basis for both partners to incorporate MS. The best thing is for both of you to agree, as far as you are able, that you are going to work together to come to terms with MS. Neither of you can afford to deny its existence and its impact on your relationship – no relationship works well if reality is ignored.

Next, it is vital to improve communication with each other. While it will also be important to communicate with other people and gain their support, the most important relationship is the one with your partner. Communicating well is tough, and there is always room for improvement. It is worthwhile to seek advice and learn new skills. There are books to consult, professionals to talk to and courses available on how to improve the way you relate to others. Good communication is the best antidote to an ailing relationship. Once you start working together on that, you will find yourselves able to deal with difficulties frankly, handle conflict constructively, and to seek new options when the old ways are no longer practicable.

Whether or not you have MS, one of the most difficult things in a relationship is to dare to be the person you are, to accept that you do not have to be different, that you can feel what you feel, take the space you need to thrive in and ask for your needs to be met. Because you need acceptance and fear rejection, you can easily slip into the position of covering up your needs and inadequacies. To be honest and open about them may sound a tall order, but it is a worthwhile goal. It puts the responsibility on you first to know yourself, and then to invite your partner to respond. It is important to emphasize that your partner always has the right to say that he or she can meet some, a few or none of your needs at any given time. You have the same right. The value of expressing your needs and feelings is not to demand that they be fulfilled, but to communicate them honestly in an unthreatening way. If you both know what is going on, you can make an honest response and face up to the consequences, without having to spend time imagining what the other is thinking and feeling. Trying to 'mind read' is impossible anyway, and eats up anxious hours.

One of the things that upsets good communication in a relationship is not being able to express your true feelings. This is not easy for most people at the best of times, and when MS is part of the scene it is particularly difficult. Feelings and fears of dependency cause extra strains in the relationship which can result in feelings of anger, fear and sadness. If these emotions are not expressed but bottled up, then you may find a distance developing between you and your partner. Deprived of closeness you may experience rejection, you may deny or over-protect, you may manipulate and you may feel guilty.

Sometimes this can escalate to a point where your relationship gets damaged or destroyed. Alternatively, one or both of you may find the strain so great that you want to take it out on the other – or yourself – and may behave in an anti-social, self-destructive way, such as taking to drink. A few will contemplate suicide. If any of these reactions become part of your relationship, you need to take stock of what is happening and get help to resolve them. Counselling will help you to face your feelings and work them through.

The most explosive feeling is anger – a very common emotion in MS relationships, but one rarely admitted to. Anger is a natural reaction when you are frustrated in your attempts to achieve a goal. You may bottle up your frustrations until you become tense and unable to share them easily. You are crowded in by them, and experience unpleasant negative reactions to others, especially your partner. You can find yourself exploding with frustration when you feel you should be able to achieve something very simple and can't, and similar feelings are experienced if your partner suggests even mildly that you should do something you sense you cannot do. It is frustrating not to be able to do what you used to do so easily. It does take time to adjust to limitations, and it takes time too to find new ways round the blocks. It is only by venting the frustration without violence that you can release the energy of the anger and focus on other options and activities.

It is noticeable how often tense, angry feelings are experienced before an MS exacerbation. You may not be conscious of physical feelings of ill-ease, and may interpret them in a psychological way because your irritability interferes with your relationship. It is almost as if you are searching for a psychological explanation of vague physical sensations still in the background, unable yet to accept the reality of hidden symptoms until they emerge fully. In the meantime, your body is already reacting and under tension. It takes very little then to trigger an outburst of angry feelings. (People react in a similar way when they are coming down with a cold.) Thus it helps if you and your partner can keep a weather eye open to this hidden cause of anger or irritability. It is physiologically based, in part, and does not deserve to be made an issue of.

There is a good side to anger, and that is when you can channel the frustrations you feel about MS into constructive and creative outlets. Anger does not have to be expressed in damaging ways, but can push you and your partner into doing something worthwhile. It's the good anger that energizes you to take part in a backgammon marathon, do a parachute jump, organize a charity fashion show or sit in your wheelchair and collect funds for MS research and welfare.

If you live with a chronic illness it is likely to have some effect on your personality, because you put up with it day in and day out. If your chronic illness is a neurological one like MS, the neurological damage may result in a further impact on your personality. Demyelination in MS can interfere with your emotions, your mental faculties, your memory and your concentration. The lesions causing this may have a permanent effect or simply produce temporary fluctuations, so the effect on your personality may either be very subtle or so pronounced it could be taken for bloody-mindedness. You may not realize there is any change in you, but your partner may become aware that you are undergoing a slight change in character – in much the same way that too much alcohol has an effect. He or she needs to understand that your MS can exaggerate what you are feeling. You may feel low and depressed or unusually bright and cheerful in the face of adversity. Your MS may affect your ability to think straight and reason soundly. You may feel out of balance with yourself, as if you were only partially in control. It's a lot for one body to cope with, and if as a result you turn in on yourself or become more self-centred than usual, your partner may misread this as your being selfish. You may not realize that at such times you become abrasive, critical and insensitive, to the point of hurting others and yourself – but your partner will. He or she may want to confront you about the way your attitude has changed, if it is negative, and try to make you change back again. If the change is due to MS, there is a limit to how much you can do until the inflammation causing the exacerbation passes. It is best not to take too much notice of it. It becomes a more worrying problem if MS has a permanent and negative effect on your personality. It is so hard to remember to blame the MS, not the person, who needs special understanding and love.

Because MS symptoms so often limit what you can and cannot do, you may find yourself forced into new roles in a relationship. This may have a disruptive effect. It is humiliating no longer to be able to do what you have previously counted important and pleasurable. It is frustrating for your partner not to be able to rely on you for certain things either. Not being able to work, get about independently or maintain a satisfying sexual relationship in the way you used to are bound to result in feelings of tension and guilt until both of you have had time to adjust. But being forced to change the nature of your role in a relationship is not an insurmountable barrier, and need never be used as an excuse to break up. It is good to give yourself and your partner space to try on 'new hats', experimenting to see how best the two of you can cope together. Your partner may sometimes be concerned to help you strike a balance between what you can manage to do and how realistic it is to exert that amount of energy on achieving it. This can become quite a crucial issue during exacerbations, relapses, and longer spells of disabling symptoms. It helps if you can talk over your priorities together, and assess what your energy level and physical skills are. Since the latter vary with MS, it is your priorities that need checking to see whether they are still viable.

This became an issue for Eileen while she was getting over an attack and could not face having people round. Before, she had had such a reputation for serving up delicious dinners of mouth-watering home-made food. Now she wasn't well enough to do any of that, she always found some excuse not to entertain. Yet she and her husband needed to meet friends in their own home sometimes, the way they previously had. It was only after friends began dropping in unexpectedly and simple basket meals were rustled up with everyone's help that Eileen began to see her real priority was being able to welcome guests to the relaxed atmosphere of the home. With her husband's help she became clear what her priority in entertaining was, and together they found alternative ways of having guests round. She said she had felt very guilty about the whole situation. It took her a long time to accept that since she was not responsible for having MS, she did not need to feel guilty anymore.

Some of the symptoms of MS threaten independence. But while it is hard to accept that disability and relapses may force you to be dependent on your partner and others for physical care, it is important to distinguish between having to be dependent because you are unable to do certain things (washing, feeding and so on) and remaining independent as a person in your own right. If you feel you are being 'done to' rather than 'doing', it is easy to slip into becoming dependent on your partner and letting feelings of dependency grow. This upsets the equality of your relationship. On the other hand, if you fear losing your independence, you may so fight against it that you never let your partner do anything to help you, even when it would be normal and natural to do so. It is hardest to accept that sickness and disability may force you to rely on others for physical care. You may be shy or embarrassed about your natural body functions when you need help in getting washed, going to the toilet or being attended to during a menstrual period. Every relationship is different in its balance of dependence and independence, and there is always room for you to discover what is most appropriate for you and your partner now. The most natural person to turn to is usually your partner, and after that to a professional carer such as a nurse.

Your partner may feel uncomfortable or reluctant to nurse you this way on a regular basis. This does not mean your partner does not care, but rather that he or she finds nursing care difficult. There are, in fact, long-term advantages to getting as much professional help as possible, as it helps you and your partner to maintain a more intimate and loving relationship. Your sexual relationship as an equal can be impaired if your partner permanently takes over the role of nurse rather than lover. What counts with MS is your ability to remain your own person and to relate to others, and it is this that will allow you and your partner to grow together. When Tom insisted on struggling through the snow from the house to the car with a walking-frame one bitter winter, he nearly got frostbite, but gained nothing else. Using a wheelchair was quicker, warmer, lost him no dignity and gave him energy to enjoy being out with his partner.

There is a fine line between being cared for on your terms and being smothered with unwanted attention. If your partner is the sort of person who cares for you too readily when you can manage reasonably well yourself, it may be that he or she is responding to his or her own needs and not yours. He or she may be compensating for what are perceived to be your disadvantages. You may even feel you are being hurried along into permanent disability. The end result is a relationship based on domination, in which your partner gets the upper hand, so to speak, by pushing you to accept a dependent role. You are discouraged from doing anything much yourself, no longer believe you can, and may feel resentful. Jenni's husband was the model of a caring husband and did everything for her. His sudden death left her helpless but in time she discovered she could manage on her own and enjoyed being able to look after herself. Smothering has no place in a good relationship.

Occasionally, a partner chooses to ignore any information about MS in general and your MS in particular, in some extreme cases by burying his or her head in the sand and being unpleasantly surly with it. Such a partner wants to make it clear that MS changes nothing in your relationship, and just doesn't want to know. Partners like this are either totally inconsiderate and selfish, or too hurt to be supportive. They cope by denying reality, and leave you feeling utterly rejected and depressed. Such extremes are rare, but far commoner are partners who side-step involvement with MS whenever possible, hoping that in time it will go away provided you don't mention it again. They shut their ears when anyone tries to tell them about the invisible symptoms of MS, especially fatigue.

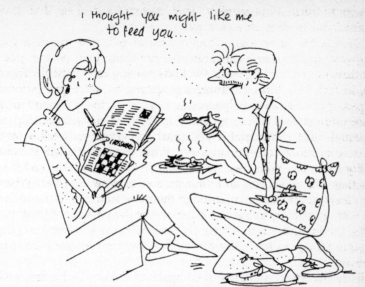

I thought you might like me to feed you....

IF YOUR PARTNER IS THE SORT OF PERSON WHO CARES FOR YOU TOO READILY WHEN YOU CAN MANAGE REASONABLY WELL YOURSELF....

They ignore any warnings you give about how much it can hurt to be touched when you are suffering from impaired sensation, or what pain you suffer from being jolted about in a wheelchair because they won't learn to handle one properly. Such insensitivity and denial place intolerable stresses on a relationship. Your options are to put up with it or to get out quick.

Each partner is responsible for maintaining a relationship. In the new situation, with MS, you can both choose to grow together in a special closeness or struggle in a mesh of conflict. Take time to re-evaluate what you are willing to give to your partner and decide what is realistic. It is important to seek help whenever necessary, for there are times when an impartial outsider with the right skills is a better source of support for you both. To dare to explore new options can result in a most rewarding and exciting life together.

Coping with children

It is sometimes said that when one member of the family becomes ill, the whole family is affected. That effect need not be negative – it can be a positive, wholesome one. With MS you can still be a parent who passes on, in the caring and considerate way that counts, the lessons in life that matter most, as well as values and skills to last a lifetime. No parent can give more than he or she received and experienced, and MS, for all its disadvantages, does force you to take stock – an extra, enriching experience the value of which can be easily overlooked. A parent with MS often worries that his or her children will be missing out on proper care and attention, outings, the rough and tumble of games and family fun. There is some truth in this, but it does not mean that their upbringing will be any less adequate than the average. Children are highly practical, and if given adequate information they understand quickly what you can and cannot do. They have a right to know what MS means in language they understand, so they can make sense of what's going on. They often become more anxious when they are denied knowledge about what you are experiencing, or about any hospital visits or tests you need. Far from shielding them from MS, you are exposing them to it. Their natural sensitivity may enable them to pick up what is implied but left unsaid, or they may jump to conclusions more alarming than reality. There will be times to involve them in major family decisions so they don't feel excluded and resentful. Sometimes they take the blame for the way you behave because of MS, and suppose that they are a burden. You may be the sort who soldiers on past your fatigue level until you find yourself getting ratty and snapping at them. Your mood swings then intensify as you push yourself over the top trying to prove you are a 'normal' parent. There are children who believe their bad behaviour may have caused you to have an attack; they may even start to feel guilty for having been born. It may be a fact that your MS symptoms appeared after your child's birth, but remember to give reassurance that he or she wasn't responsible for their appearance.

Children tend to go one of two ways: they either seek to separate themselves from their MS parent or both parents, or they throw themselves into helping like 'little adults'. Some are embarrassed to be seen out with a disabled parent. They may express their envy of their friends whose parents don't have MS, in much the same way as some poor kids envy rich ones. This is hurtful, but a common reaction at a certain age and for certain personalities. Sometimes the fact that a parent can't do something the way other mothers and fathers can gets blown out of all proportion. It is sad when a father who's loved kicking a ball about with his children can no longer do so, and yet it needn't spell disaster in their relationship. What children are often really reacting to when they seem to fuss about not having a footballer of a dad is the unspoken self-blame and disappointment of the parent. Perhaps your children are taking their cue from you. If you can admit your disappointment, accept it, and move on to emphasize the positive aspects of your relationship, your child will feel he has gained from you and not lost. Other children are very protective, and find ways of speaking out about MS so that their friends and neighbours understand better.

It is one thing to encourage your children to do additional household chores within reason, but it is quite another to lean on them for emotional support and comfort. They are your children, and it is always your responsibility to be available as much as possible to care for and make adequate provision for them. Children are very accommodating and help willingly if they know they are really loved. Their respect for you must never be abused by trying to get them to side with you and take on an adult role to fight for you. It is essential that you develop a network of other supports – family, friends, doctors, nurses and paramedics, social workers, clergymen, the local branch of a society concerned with MS or general disability problems (for addresses, see page 140), and other people with MS. These are the proper sources of adult support, and not your children.

Coping with parents

Parents of someone with MS often feel in some way responsible. They will admit to a niggling fear that they may have passed on MS, although there's no medical evidence of a direct genetic link. They will also wonder if they failed to protect you from something in the environment that may have caused MS.

It is understandable that they are concerned and wish to do what they can to help. They may well be able to offer support in very practical ways by being there to listen and comfort, baby-sitting, assisting with household chores and gardening, accompanying you shopping and on trips out if that is what you want to do together. Their help may be invaluable if given sensitively and unobtrusively. As with your partner, much depends on the quality of your relationship with your parents before you were diagnosed, and how ready you are to initiate any changes that are needed.

There are some parents who find it difficult to accept MS even when it is staring them in the face. It is as if they cannot accept that their child could ever have anything wrong. This attitude, which places high priority on keeping the side up and achieving well, is one a child may also have shared unquestioningly. It is an attitude in which anything less than perfection – and illness comes into this bracket – is seen as failure. Unfortunately, this sort of attitude frequently stands in the way of coming to terms with MS.

It is not uncommon to discover that you are clinging on to values and opinions about illness and disability which you learnt at home as the norm but which your new experience with MS demands you should confront. It does not help you at all if you persist in believing that having MS is somehow a sign of personal failure. Mavis's parents obviously felt this way about her, and were helpless to make any meaningful contact with their 40-year-old daughter. Like a little girl she went through a phase of apparently trying to please them and everyone else as though to compensate for her MS. Far from getting her the understanding and support she so desperately needed, it only alienated her from her parents even more. The important factor for her and many others with a similar experience is that her previous relationship with her parents had never been that good, and she had always been the one who tried to compensate for the shortfall. As a child she had never succeeded in getting the unconditional love she craved. Now that an MS diagnosis made her feel vulnerable, she needed support herself and her parents didn't know how to give it. The only practical solution was to keep a distance between them and for Mavis to get her support elsewhere. In order to do that she needed to cut her ties and accept responsibility for herself. She had to learn she had the right to make up her own mind and choose her own priorities, especially now she had MS.

There is a danger in some families with MS that the parents will come in and virtually take over. If that is what you (and your partner) want, then it is fine. If not, it is an invasion of your privacy which you have every right to oppose.

It is hard to stand by when your own child is hurt. It would be so good to remove the hurt and make it better again. Good parents will naturally feel protective and caring, and will look for ways to help. At the same time they will often experience helplessness too, and need guidance on how to relate to you.

Coping with friends

'You certainly know who your friends are when you've got MS.' You may suddenly discover some of your friends have amazing depths of kindness, while others turn out to be the shallow, fair-weather sort. Some stick by you through thick and thin; others cool off and maintain a cordial distance for fear they may get involved more than they want to; and a few disappear fast.

The best friends are those who find out what you want and do not jump to conclusions. You have a responsibility to share with them such information about MS as will enable them to support

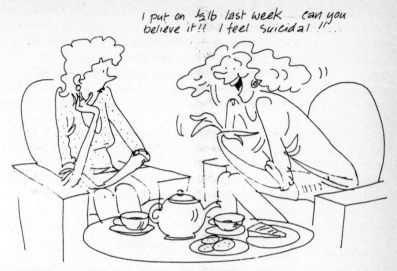

I put on ½lb last week ... can you believe it!! I feel suicidal !! ...

YOU WILL NEED TO DEAL WITH FRIENDS WHO TAKE ADVANTAGE OF THE FACT THAT YOU WILL ALWAYS BE AT HOME, SERVE DECENT TEA & COFFEE AND WILL LISTEN TO THEM.

you best. You also need to be aware that friends will vary as to how much they actually want to know. A treasured few will let you pour your heart out, and you will soon learn to choose what and how much to share with whom. Friends can only take so much, and you need to respect their limits if you want to maintain contact. You will need to learn how to deal with friends who like to organize you, who blunder but mean well, who take advantage of the fact you may always be at home, serve decent tea or coffee, and will listen to them, and those who visit you out of sympathy, to do you a good turn. If you become unable to get about easily, you will have fewer opportunities to make and keep friendships going. At times MS will curtail social life. You may be the sort of person who is afraid to say anything to hurt anyone and yet find you sometimes need to say no to a visit or outing because it is just not one of your good days. In the end, communicating your needs so that you give your friends a chance to help meet them is one of the things that keeps the friendship going. It could be a new experience to get from a relationship as much as you give, and for a while it may feel lopsided that way. It is frequently friends, rather than close members of the family, who enable us to accept that MS does not diminish us but provides a new framework to live in.

Coping with your doctor

An MS diagnosis will mark the start of a new emphasis in your relationship with your doctor. It is a good time to check if you really have the right sort of doctor, someone who is comfortable with you and your MS. The doctor–patient relationship is a professional one in which the patient is offered what he or she needs personally on professional terms. Usually it works well this way. However, when a patient feels vulnerable – and this is common with an MS diagnosis – he or she may try to change the basis of the relationship and want to make an ally of the doctor. The patient begins to expect more from the doctor than can be given professionally.

The first thing to be clear about is that no doctor, however good, will have all the answers. You can't demand more than a doctor can give, and you are certainly being completely unreasonable if you pester your doctor for detailed information about your *future* MS. What you may be doing is attacking the doctor with all the anger and resentment you have stored up because you don't want to have MS. Doctors are a common target for patients with chronic illnesses, especially MS. You may storm, rant and rave, but in the end you must accept the fact that MS is a very variable disease and no two cases are ever alike. You are the one who is largely responsible for managing your MS, and you are wise to invite your doctor to work with you.

If your doctor could be honest with you, he would probably admit that he would rather not have any MS patients on his register. Doctors are trained to cure rather than treat. It is natural they should want their patients to get better – whether from the viewpoint of compassion, wanting to alleviate suffering or from that of success, seeing their skills work.

With your MS diagnosis you present a challenge to your doctor. Doctors can offer you their full professional skills of treatment and management, and they know as well as you do that that won't always be enough. If they are blessed with the skills of good communication, effective counselling and insight, they will get close to meeting your needs as you battle to come to terms with MS. You will value your doctor for understanding that you sometimes just need to talk. You will spill out a catalogue of vague symptoms he or she can do little about, and have another go at winkling out new insights as to how you are really doing, knowing that there are no answers. All the doctor can give is tender loving care, for you both know there is no cure. Value the doctor who is able to give such care and forgive the one who is unable to. The reason for not being able to may be to do with his or her own personality, with MS in particular, or because your personalities clash.

Doctors often feel inadequate or frustrated when faced with MS patients. That is hardly surprising when they are made the target of their patients' emotional reactions – for aren't they there to let off steam at? Doctors must be careful not to take such attacks personally, telling themselves that they don't deserve this, and hoping that you will experience some relief afterwards. Few doctors have the time or skills to confront patients therapeutically and enable them to cope with the anger, bitterness, fear and sadness, and then move on to living well with MS. Some practices can refer MS patients on to counsellors or psychiatric social workers for this kind of help. Alternatively, branches of the MS Society (see page 140) offer skilled support via trained voluntary workers or self-help groups.

There is a very real problem of coping with the hidden and subjective symptoms of MS. Both before and after diagnosis some doctors are sceptical about these, often labelling them incorrectly as 'neurotic' or 'hypochondriac'. What doctors need to realize is that you may experience so many of these symptoms that those you begin by describing may be chosen almost at random, because they're the ones that have affected you most emotionally, or even because you have forgotten the others. It can be helpful to keep a list of what you want to share with your doctor. MS can make someone more prone to forgetfulness than average. Doctors need to remind themselves that their MS patients do not necessarily know what weight to attach to their symptoms, and patiently wait to hear the whole list! Getting your doctor's support and understanding over fatigue, bizarre sensations, pain and visual problems does confirm that these are recognized symptoms of MS. This is a particularly difficult area, since these symptoms could be attributed to causes other than MS, so it helps to be able to pass on information about your MS that you know is medically confirmed.

A tricky area for doctors is giving advice on the subject of diets and alternative medicine. They have a responsibility to protect their patients from quackery and opportunists out for money. They are also concerned that false hopes of a cure are not raised when the treatment on offer defies all the laws of medicine and scientific reason. They would be unprofessional if they did not warn against unlikely cures. They understand the depression that results from disillusionment when a cure does not work. On the other hand, many doctors are happy to keep an interested eye on a patient who follows some diet regime as long as they are reasonably certain it will do no harm.

The following are suggestions on how to get the best from your doctor:

● Be punctual.

- Be specific about why you are seeing him or her. A doctor needs to know if you have come for a chat, a prescription renewal, or specific help, in order to give priority to whatever is concerning you.
- Explain clearly your physical symptoms, any reactions to medication and any other concerns – in that order.
- Write down a list of questions you want to ask and jot down the answers too, in case you forget.
- Follow the advice of your doctor. Ask, if you don't understand or forget what is said.
- Be polite and generous as you share any information about yourself. You are your own expert in MS. Remember that your doctor cannot mind-read.
- Try not to become too familiar. Doctors are engaged in professional work, and are not there just because you need someone to chat to. They have a right to privacy away from the office.

MS and society

Sickness and society

A diagnosis of MS does not necessarily imply either sickness or disability. The frequent response of 'But you look so well!' indicates not only that looks belie a person's condition, at least at first glance, but also that with MS someone is clearly not sick in the conventional way.

Society tries to contain sickness by specifying certain conditions the sick should fulfil in order to get rid of the illness, so that once again, when recovered, they may resume their place. It is important to understand that society has such rules about health and sickness in order to be able to assess what is an appropriate reaction to MS.

Society's first ground-rule is that the sick should be pronounced so by doctors, withdraw to an isolated position and give up social responsibilities until health is restored. Even if your sort of MS doesn't obviously affect your lifestyle, and you believe this rule does not apply to you, there will be some people who expect you to adopt a sickness role anyway. Frequently, though, the fluctuations of MS will result in your curtailing or opting out of some responsibilities at home, work and socially. If you are determined to hold a job down at all costs, you may not have the energy to garden or go to parties. So you will withdraw in order to maintain your priorities. This may become a permanent way of life, so you need to counterbalance it with input that supports you and draws you back into contact with others.

Society's second rule for the sick is that they should be taken care of. This is only applicable during an MS relapse or when disability is severe. Apart from these times you can maintain your independence and ask for what care you need when necessary.

The third rule states that the sick should always want to get well. This probably causes most aggravation. Of course you want to be well and never again be reminded of this chronic disease. If anyone could tell you exactly what to do to be well, you'd follow that advice like a shot, which is why so many so-called treatments and cures gain such a following. How well you are on an imaginary scale of nought to ten can vary from less than one to more than eight in the space of a day, so you hesitate to commit yourself to saying how well you are feeling right now. With MS it is wiser, and more within practical reach, to aim at improving the quality of your life than to expect a return to being well.

The last ground-rule is that the sick should get the best medical advice and then follow it obediently. This is also of limited relevance, as with MS there has to be a pooling of co-operative effort between doctors, paramedics and you with your expertise on your own condition.

MS in a health-orientated society

If you have a chronic disease like MS you may not class yourself as being in good health, but neither can you necessarily claim that you are sick. You may experience spells of sickness, but the rest of the time you are either more or less aware of the fact that you have MS. You and those around you need to be clear as to whether having MS makes you a sick person or not. If it does, then you need to know how to react and what role is appropriate for you.

There seem to be three main reactions to being sick in a healthy society. Although you may not see yourself fitting any one of these caricatures completely, you will probably recognize certain tendencies in yourself.

You may be the type who at the first sign of what may pass as a symptom, however mild, fleeting and unobtrusive, rushes to a doctor for diagnosis, care and cure. You are on your guard against potential illness and determined to avoid it. You have faith in the ability of doctors to remove ill-health and expect treatment. When the cause of your health problem is MS you will soon be disillusioned, because no doctor can give you specific advice on the cause, course, prognosis or treatment of your MS that will take it away. Doctors cannot know what is as yet unknowable. They have had to come to terms with this sort of frustration over and over again in each area of their medical training and practice. It is not unique to MS but forms the barrier to knowledge in every branch of medical science. If you are potentially a doctor-dependent patient, believing that doctors should have all the answers, this is a hard reality to accept. If you cannot accept it, you will spend more time and energy on battling with doctors than on learning to live with MS.

On the other hand, you may be the sort of person who takes total responsibility for yourself right from the start. You have probably been very aware of what has been going wrong in your body and have done all you can to improve your condition. You will have checked your diet, supplemented it with additional remedies, vitamins and minerals, and chosen to focus on what you know you can achieve, turning your back on any non-essential activities. You are in control, and have decided to do it your way. You are determined to preserve the outward signs of functioning healthily in a health-valuing society. And you have MS too. You may so value remaining part of society that you overlook the real effects your MS is having on you. By the time you are willing to admit to some health problem and see a doctor, your MS will have become visibly severe and you will probably have been pushed into consulting one by family, friends or colleagues. Self-reliant, you are used to driving yourself hard and determined to keep going, but you pay a heavy price. Yours is a tight-rope of an existence in which you are maintaining the best lifestyle you can with your current health problems. It is precarious, but it means you avoid the sickness role and stay in the mainstream of society. Although you make up your own mind what your priorities are you can become so single-minded about keeping going at all costs that you neglect to ensure you have sufficient caring support from others. You need that balance.

Finally, you may be the sort of person who loves being part of society so much that you can never afford to be sick and take time off to recuperate. You will probably be aware of abnormal symptoms, but are unwilling to give up an active working and/or social life. You disregard the effects of MS by never adjusting your lifestyle, going on to the point of total exhaustion and collapse. You believe that if you make any allowance for your MS, you are somehow losing, giving in and failing. Yours is an all-or-nothing existence, with high stakes. While the going is good, you can pretend MS does not exist and enjoy the full swing of normal living. If ever your MS threatens to limit your activities and confine you away from the mainstream of society, you will struggle with the feeling that you have to shut yourself off from people. You are likely to need understanding help, and to be taught how to modify your reactions. With MS you have the right to be part of society, however highly that society values good health and feels discomforted by sickness.

Optimism versus pessimism

A natural optimist is already capitalizing on a powerful force that will help in coping better with MS, both psychologically and physically. Optimists see any problem as temporary, specific to a known cause and nothing to do with themselves. They experience a buoyancy that gives their bodies stamina to fight disease and their minds courage to explore ways of overcoming it. They can laugh at themselves and their situation. It is not that life doesn't deal out some blows, but if you are an optimist you are better equipped to ride them.

If you are a dyed-in-the-wool pessimist, you will limit your body's rehabilitation by your negative thoughts. Changing them is difficult, and demands determination – and, in most cases, professional help. You will need to talk to someone like a counsellor, therapist or clergyman who understands and has skills to help you become more positive. Remember, MS gives you good reason to initiate changes.

Control

The issue of control is especially pertinent to MS as well as to other diseases that strike at random and without warning. You are suddenly knocked off your feet – literally, as well as figuratively – and experience what it is like not to be in control of what is happening to you. This is very frightening, and your panic can spread to other areas of your life before it takes the time it needs to subside.

Once you begin to accept you are still valuable as a person even if your body does not always function the way you would like, you begin to be in control of your own life and destiny again. Some people find a religious faith or philosophy of life helps them to achieve this. Others seek some sort of professional help from counsellors or therapists. Once in control, you experience freedom to grow as a person looking for options, experimenting, always moving on. The disease may still be beyond your control in a medical sense, but you don't let it stifle who you are and what you want to do.

Some people use MS as a perfect excuse to control others and their environment. They have failed to accept a change of control in themselves with MS, so they concentrate their controlling powers elsewhere. Ruth was a prime example of a controlling lady. She sat back in her chair and directed the household from there. She had

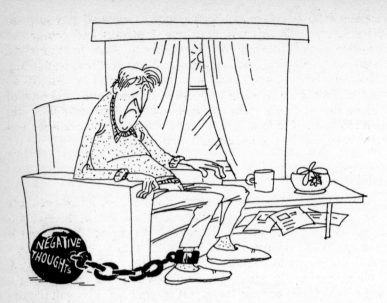

IF YOU ARE A DYED-IN-THE-WOOL PESSIMIST, YOU WILL LIMIT THE BODY'S REHABILITATION BY YOUR NEGATIVE THOUGHTS...

everyone running at her beck and call. Her attention to detail was meticulous, and home-helps soon learnt to replace ornaments in the exact spot after dusting. Her controlling attitude extended to her family and friends. It gave her a sort of power to insist things be done her way, but not a gentleness and warmth that attracted people to her or gave her happiness in living. While you have a right to take control of your own life, you have no right to trample over the rights of others.

Attitudes

'It's your attitude that counts' is a statement that can get under your skin and itch. If pronounced like a challenge, it can sound a damning one. It seems to suggest that a simple change of attitude would rid us of any difficulty with MS and perhaps even remove it permanently.

MS gives you a fresh opportunity to rethink opinions, values and stances from a new vantage point. You will soon become aware of your attitude towards yourself, towards sickness, towards disability in general and MS in particular. The attitudes of society at large and people you know will come across loud and clear, and may surprise and shock you. It will take you time, frankness and courage to challenge any of these attitudes if you have to. Attitude can make a difference to physical, mental, emotional and spiritual well-being. You do not have to get it right all at once, but people with MS do need to get started as early as possible on developing the type of outlook that will help them live well with MS. It is possible to win with MS and not to lose. It is never too late to look for options and make changes. This is the attitude that counts.

Accepting MS

Living well with MS means accepting it has moved in with you. It's a bit like fitted furniture, so permanently there that in the end you do not notice it. MS may be something you cannot escape but it need not be threatening. You do not have to welcome it like a friend, but you cannot ignore it either. MS must be accommodated.

When you finally agree to accommodate it, you are entering a pact in which you become the expert on your MS. You will require information about the disease and support from many sources but you must take responsibility for yourself now and in the future. MS may scream, shout and throw tantrums but it doesn't have to take over. You give it houseroom, but on your terms.

Strategy of coping

In coping, there are basically three ways of management. The first is to plan ahead right now while you have time and energy to build up the resources you will need for what lies ahead. It is a management strategy in which you anticipate the future, putting by for a rainy day. Given the fact of your MS, what are you likely to need in the future to help you to cope as well as possible? Only you know what resources you would like to develop within yourself. Certainly, with a disease like MS it really helps to learn how to be at peace with the person you are. Some people find this possible through relaxation classes, meditation or a faith.

It also helps when you have MS to find ways of maintaining your dignity as a person who knows what you want and is able to ask for it straight. It is therefore important to learn how to make decisions well, and to learn to feel at ease in your relationships with other people. Whatever enables you to be in control of who you are and how well you relate to others can improve your quality of life, a quality you hold of value when MS moves in.

There is also some practical forward planning you may wish to consider. For example, if you are thinking of moving house, you may be wise to consider whether to choose a home with easy access for a wheelchair, and one that has a downstairs cloakroom. Forward planning is an immensely practical skill in the process of coping.

The second management strategy in coping is the skill of cushioning yourself. You can do this by denying or ignoring what is happening because to face up to its cold reality is more than you can handle at that time. Another way of doing this is to count your blessings. MS may be affecting you badly enough but you are prepared to admit openly that there are people who are worse off. It is inevitable with a disease like MS that there will be black times physically and psychologically when, as it were, you need to go into neutral and coast along for a while. This isn't a time to sort things out but to be snuggled and cosseted around with cushions and let time pass. You can pick up whatever concerns you at a later time, when you feel strong enough to deal with it again.

The third way which you can choose to manage a crisis is by facing up to the facts. It is a constructive strategy which involves you in becoming fully aware of what is actually happening to you right here and now. It is a strategy that demands you take responsibility for the way you react, feel and think. It works to the extent that you reach out for support from others who care about you.

You will need to make use of each of these coping strategies at different times. It doesn't matter so much whether your attempts to cope are successful or not. It is the trying that counts, and this has its own positive spin-off.

Helplessness

There will be times when you feel helpless. It may be because you are physically helpless, dependent on others to care for you, or needing much more practical help to cope with daily life. On the other hand it could be that you have reached a low ebb emotionally and feel drained of all resources. Living with fatigue and other MS symptoms can become wearisome at times, and it is natural to respond by wondering whether or not you have the resources to pull through. At times like these you are likely to feel helpless. It is a feeling that will pass in its own time. It is important not to panic when you feel helpless, but to accept it is a temporary imbalance.

What can happen is that you pay too much attention to these feelings of helplessness. Instead of accepting them as feelings you may experience for a little while but gradually recover from as you gain in strength, find your symptoms easing or just get used to the new state of affairs, you may fall into the trap of paying too much attention to them. If you allow yourself to indulge in pessimism and feed off the helplessness, you will soon find yourself stuck in a negative way of thinking. This will discolour the whole of your life. It will make you prone to repeated spells of mild depression, and you may even find yourself wanting to chuck it all in and accept a submissive exit from life. This was Dorothy's experience. She believed she had lost a psychological battle with herself, and as a result felt out of control of her own life. Her deep sense of helplessness made her think her MS symptoms were worse than they really were. In her helplessness, she behaved in character with her feelings; she neglected her health, didn't eat properly, and found she wasn't sleeping well. She isolated herself from the support of family, friends and doctor.

Recent research with cancer patients has shown that feelings of helplessness and end-of-the-road pessimism may actually hamper the immune system. This factor is also likely to be significant in MS. It is not feeling helpless for a while that matters. It is remaining helpless, and no longer believing you can do anything to change it that really knocks you back.

Stress and MS

Stress is one of those inevitable concomitants of modern life, and much talked about in negative terms. However, stress isn't only negative. It comes in a variety of guises, and in a positive light can act as a challenge that forces you to change or make adjustments. Stress gives purpose to what you do, but you can also get too much of even a good thing. Stress becomes negative when you dig in your heels and fail to make the adjustments required. Confront stress with refusal to act and there's a difficult time ahead. It is not really stress that is the problem but the way you handle it. The key is your ability to adjust to or cope with stress.

Events that have a stressful effect include many everyday experiences such as moving house, getting married and having a baby, all of which are associated with pleasure and fun too. Exams, tensions at work and taking on new responsibilities are stresses that are part of a lifestyle accepted by many. Conflict within close relationships, divorce, unemployment, accidents, severe illness and death bring stress everyone would rather avoid. Each stressful event has a physical, emotional and/or social effect.

There is no doubt that stress has a direct effect on health because of the way you perceive it. The extent of its effect depends on how long the stress lasts, how intensely it is experienced, and, most significantly, on how susceptible as an individual you are to it. Your personality, coupled with the support you need, determines how

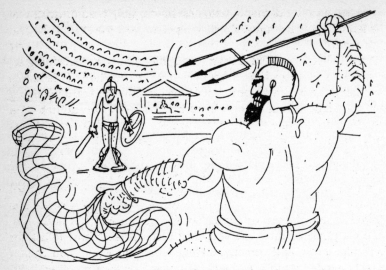

CONFRONT STRESS WITH A REFUSAL TO ACT AND
THERE'S A DIFFICULT TIME AHEAD!

you view stress. Stressful situations can provoke you to anger so that you fight back, or else you feel fear and want to run away and avoid it all. The most dangerous reactions to stress are feelings of hopelessness and helplessness. When you feel unable to cope for a period of time, your body is more likely to give abnormal or lowered immune responses. This can precipitate the appearance of symptoms and the onset of disease. Many body mechanisms react negatively to a helpless reaction to stress. It makes good sense, then, once you have MS, to check that you are giving yourself the best chance, and to learn how to cope with stress well.

There is some evidence that many people with MS have experienced three times the normal number of stressful life events in a two-year period prior to early MS symptoms appearing. Poor handling of these stresses perhaps helps trigger MS. Once you have MS, the way you deal with even temporary stress may precipitate exacerbations, so you need to take stock and check you are developing skilful ways of coping with stress.

Accepting help

Most people need to feel independent and in control. With MS the problem comes when a person runs out of energy, skills and initiative and really does need help from others. It is difficult then to request and not demand. Often asking for help is so difficult that it is left until the last minute, when a person is at the lowest ebb and least tactful.

Another fear that comes from accepting help, is that by doing so, you may feel placed in a socially inferior position. It is not a question of being ungrateful, but of the difficulty in acknowledging that you stand out as being different and needy. You do not want pity. You do not like to admit you are not able to do certain things for yourself. You may even suspect that others will be glad of an opportunity to demonstrate how caring they are.

You are happy to accept help when you need it and not just because someone sees you are disabled and assumes you cannot manage. You need to learn not to devalue yourself because help is offered or not offered, or because of the way in which it is offered.

To get past this dilemma you must yourself learn how to ask for help, pleasantly and directly, stating what you want. You cannot expect anyone to mind-read what you want. By treating others with directness and respect you will make it possible for them to treat you that way too.

Disability

Reactions to disability

When MS symptoms interfere with your lifestyle, you clearly have a problem with disability. It may be a disability that shows, and that others are already very aware of. Or perhaps it is a hidden disability that causes some embarrassment, such as an incontinence problem which could be managed quite discreetly with the right advice and protection. It may be a disability that could be described as an exaggeration of what everyone feels from time to time – unutterable weariness to the point of tears.

People react to disability by either hiding it or revealing all. You may be expert at brushing aside the genuine interest of others in your disability problem. Perhaps you are afraid of a flood of uncontrollable feelings sweeping over you once you start to talk about your symptoms and experience. You have to be with a safe and understanding person who asks at the right time and in the right way, or else it just is not worth the agony. Or you may keep quiet because you are ashamed of your disability. It makes you feel inferior. It is a known fact that those with a disability experience a distorted body image. They see themselves reshaped by the disability they are most aware of. It is like looking in a hall of mirrors at a fun-fair. They may also suffer from a psychological distortion which makes them believe that disability confers an inferior status.

Some people, however, want to talk about their disabilities again and again. It is as though their experience and its impact on their lives is not quite real. Talking it out and being understood brings a tremendous relief. It helps them to accept, and gives comfort and courage to go on. For them, silence may impose an intolerable stress and lead to depression.

Another reaction is to fight MS disability doggedly and seem-ingly refuse to learn to live with it. You desperately cling on to what you know as normality. You cannot accept there is no cure, but hang on, blinkered until the day comes when the answer to the MS puzzle is found and then you will step right back into normal life. Why should you make changes in the way you see yourself and live your life if later on it will turn out to have been quite unnecessary?

You may struggle with the belief that you always have to fight back against all odds to be awarded even half a place in society. Others will find that difficult to accept because although society values independence, autonomy and self-reliance, it also expects the disabled to be dependent. Your MS fluctuates anyway, and add to this the fatigue factor and it's hardly surprising that you often feel in conflict with yourself. You go to extremes – at one occasion you can be excessively normal, and at the next excessively disabled. Others must be as confused as you are.

The disability trap

The way you react to MS disability does not always relate to how severe the disease appears to be. Some are devastated by minimal symptoms and handicap, while others with severe disability take it all in their stride. Responses are very individual and depend on personality, preference of lifestyle, work and the support of others. Megan, who has never been an outdoor type and whose legs are now partially paralysed, does not hanker to roam the hills but is quite comfortable relaxing with a book or watching TV. Her disability fits easily with her interests and preferences. Accommo-dating another MS disability, though, such as eyesight problems, would be quite a different matter.

If you have mild or invisible symptoms and would pass as not disabled in any way, you may still find yourself under considerable strain and difficulty in coming to terms with MS. If a disability is obvious, everyone makes allowances for it, giving it a wide berth. Whenever you use a wheelchair you take on a new role or identity which others see as permanent. Move from the wheelchair to an ordinary chair in a restaurant and you will experience a change of attitude from those serving you. Get out of your wheelchair to stretch your legs and walk a bit in a department store and your ability to make use of a wheelchair as and when needed will cause some to take a second look and scratch their heads in confusion. Remain in your wheelchair and ask directly for what you want and you will find some people visibly surprised that wheelchairs can contain human beings who are lucid, intelligent, pleasant and have a sense of humour. It is not easy to strike a balance between hiding your disability and pushing it to the fore. You have the right to choose how you want to come across.

Choosing support

It is possible that you have never really asked for support for yourself before. You may have been the one who has always supported others and never been taken care of yourself. Your biggest struggle in learning to live with MS may be allowing yourself the right to receive support.

It is best to get an early start and begin at once experimenting with ways of being supported on your terms. You will need to be prepared to gently reject any moves by others towards being taken over. You will also need to guard against becoming demanding and fussy, and instead give others the respect you would also enjoy. Look at the way you are asking to be supported. Are you claiming rights as compensation because you have been dealt such a blow by MS? Or is yours a genuine and open request for support, made in the belief that the other has the right to say no or suggest an alternative?

You may find yourself in the midst of a power struggle with yourself and potential supporters. If you are afraid of being taken over, you may fight to remain independent at all costs. Remember you have the right to support – practical or otherwise – but not at the expense of others thinking for you. You get what you ask for, with safeguards and limits of your own choosing. You are responsible for yourself.

It helps to accept you have needs beyond the practicalities of life, needs for the attention and care you always deserve, with or without MS. There are people around you to provide that kind of support too. They may be members of your family, friends, or neighbours who spontaneously reach out to assure you they care and will stand by you regardless. Treasure them. Or they may be professional carers whose warmth and personal concern shines through their work. Both groups form the basis of your support network. With their support you know you are fulfilled and living for a purpose.

Taking responsibility
Caring for yourself

- Make sure you live well, getting the best food, short but regular periods of exercise, and all the relaxation and sleep you need.
- Cut out all non-essential activity.
- Move out of over-drive, decelerate, and idle in 'neutral' when you need to. Strike a balance between doing too little and too much.
- Learn to pace yourself and be flexible.
- Ask for the help and support you need.
- Follow the medical advice you ask for, and try any reasonable medication, treatment or therapy offered. Believe in yourself.
- Find reasons for living by creating interests.

Caring about the way you feel

- Learn to be aware of what you feel.
- Learn how to express your feelings without hurting others.
- Choose to have positive feelings.
- Learn to face up to negative feelings and let them go.
- Avoid damaging emotional stress.
- Don't isolate yourself emotionally.
- Seek the support of others who understand.

Caring about the way you see life

- Become aware of the changes you are experiencing.
- Believe change is possible and can be positive.
- Positive thinking can replace negative thinking.
- Learn how to deal with problems well by breaking them down into steps and setting a series of goals.
- Focus on the present and the future, not on the past and the present.
- Prepare yourself to cope with the effects of MS on your life and relationships.
- Plan to substitute new activities for old ones.
- Develop talents you have a use for *now*.
- Believe you will achieve a sense of peace and happiness when you come to accept the reality of MS.
- Take hold of the support a meaningful faith or philosophy of life offers.
- Choose what you want.

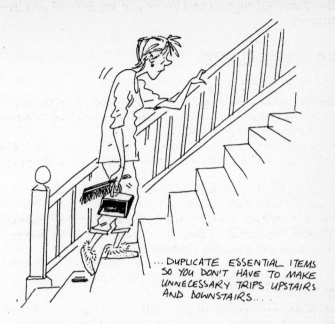

...DUPLICATE ESSENTIAL ITEMS
SO YOU DON'T HAVE TO MAKE
UNNECESSARY TRIPS UPSTAIRS
AND DOWNSTAIRS....

Caring for the practicalities of life

- Get the difficult jobs done early in the day or when you have most energy.
- If you have got a busy time ahead, rest beforehand and afterwards.
- Use holidays to relax in.
- Check that the temperature suits you where you live and work.
- Bathe in warm or tepid water.
- Keep noise and stress to a minimum.
- Use a stick, walker or wheelchair when you need to.
- Duplicate essential items so you don't have to make unnecessary trips upstairs and downstairs.
- Vary what you do so you don't strain one set of muscles.
- Take safety precautions – for instance, don't pick up heavy objects you can't carry, or handle hot things if you are not sensitive to heat, and don't fill cups to the brim.

4

Coping with the crises of MS

What turns a situation into a crisis? Is it what happens or the way we respond to what goes on? I would suggest the latter. Some people will experience the so-called crises of MS written about in this chapter calmly, accepting each as simply another of life's challenges. Others may be devastated. Everyone has a different crisis threshold – either they can take anything without batting an eyelid or the slightest thing out of the ordinary throws them. People are all different.

A crisis throws you off balance. While it lasts, you are neither winning nor losing but wavering in between. What some people call a crisis may not be one for others, but that shouldn't make them distrust their own reactions. A crisis is a situation in which you feel vulnerable and at risk in some way. You are the only one who can decide what constitutes a crisis for you. The natural reaction to the threat of crisis is to try and get back to feeling at ease again. You try out various ways of coping so that you can win through. When you find something that works, you are back on your feet again, your balance restored and the former crisis is put in the past.

Some crises seem to escalate until they appear too big to handle. It's interesting to watch how this happens. Initially people start off by coping with a crisis in the usual ways, ways that have worked in the past. If it doesn't go away, they begin to feel tense and somewhat helpless. They discover no one else has a ready-made solution that suits their crisis and so they are left to trial and error solutions that they have never used before. If none of these works, they feel extremely tense and very threatened. This is an emergency and drastic emergency measures are called for.

Some of these emergency measures may have already been useful in coming to terms with MS. One approach to take is to change goals or aspirations. Instead of insisting on becoming a top footballer when you have a gammy MS leg that won't kick, you can choose a different career that doesn't depend for its success on that leg.

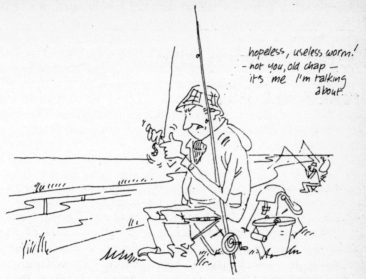

YOU MAY NEED TO CONSIDER HOW FAIR YOU ARE BEING
WHEN YOU BLAME YOURSELF FOR NOT BEING ABLE
TO DO SOMETHING LIKE TYING BAIT ON A FISH-HOOK...

Another approach is to look at the problem differently. It may be necessary to consider how fair it is to blame yourself for not being able to do something like tying bait on a fish-hook because you have MS. Why not give yourself a break, grieve or get angry, and in the breathing space that follows allow yourself to see another side to the problem. Finally you could choose to largely ignore the problem because it can't be solved as a whole, focusing on solving just part of it.

Occasionally people become so tense over a crisis and so threatened, that it all becomes too much and something has to snap. They reach breaking point and collapse into deep depression, usually accompanied by a worsening of MS symptoms. This is the time for action by the medical profession, who will use a variety of means such as tranquillizers, antidepressants, a stay in hospital, counselling, psychotherapy or psychiatric care, to help restore a state of balance.

The crisis process

A crisis such as an accident, unemployment, death, an MS diagnosis or a new MS symptom is a shock to the system. It is difficult to believe it's really going on and in disbelief you experience a sense of numbness. You need to pinch yourself to believe it is real.

After the shock and numbness you react in one of two ways – denial or outcry. Denying MS means shutting your ears to the facts given to you by doctors, ignoring what others say in confirmation of the diagnosis and minimizing your own experience. You hear only what you want to hear, and search around for an alternative that gives some hope. At times you can lose sight of reality. The mind goes round and round in circles, over the same old ground but nothing changes.

Crying out against MS is a way of saying you feel victimized. It isn't fair and you don't deserve it. It is so easy to be quick to blame others and seethe with anger. You may feel full of energy and either buzz around on a high or hold on to it and look visibly tense.

After the denial or the outcry comes the experience of loss. Losses deserve to be grieved for as it is only then that a value can be put on what you once had and it becomes possible to move ahead to a fresh start. Loss is best gone through by allowing time and space for real crying. This helps release the tension. Finally you come to the point where you can see that what you are doing to yourself isn't helpful. At this point of exhaustion or panic comes the blessing of calm insight. All is not lost and hope lies ahead.

It is now time to find out what is really going on, take a critical look at the situation and consider the options. This is when it helps to consider the opinions of others, so you have as much information as possible at your fingertips. That way you can decide what to do for the best.

Some people find it too difficult to tackle a crisis and refuse to go any further. They decide for many reasons that they are unable to take any action. It may be argued that they are overwhelmed by too many difficulties or their worsening MS makes it impossible for them to do any more, but mostly the reason lies within themselves. They would need strengthened inner resources and extra special support and care from others to go any further. They seek refuge instead in drink, drugs or self-pity which compounds the crisis. It is a tragedy that they cannot step out of the crisis but stay swallowed up in it, existing rather than living.

To live well with MS, it is necessary to go right through the crisis process until you find your way again ... a new way to step out and on. In this chapter the focus will be on some aspects of MS which are common causes of crisis.

Incontinence

For a symptom that can be treated with success or managed well, incontinence is a problem that is often blown out of proportion. Elaine, a nurse, dreaded it more than any other symptom, a fear stemming back to her own toilet-training as a child. It became such a bogey in her mind that she worked herself down into a state of gloomy depression and introversion. What she needed was reassurance that if she ever did experience incontinence problems, she could rely on a wealth of expertise to help her cope.

The fact that many people are embarrassed by bodily functions, like going to the toilet, cannot be dismissed. It is one of those natural activities people easily learn to be unnatural about. It helps not to be prudish. People have no problem accepting that babies are incontinent but often fuss and fret when emotional problems, accidents, disease or old age result in an incontinence problem in someone past babyhood. Incontinence is a very widespread problem, especially for women, but in genteel society it is a topic one would rather not mention. Even among women with MS, 20 per cent can blame their incontinence on something other than the disease. Those who suffer from it, for whatever reason, do continue to lead normal active lives once they have received treatment or been given adequate methods of coping with it.

Bladder control

What is incontinence? It is the passing of urine when you don't plan to because there is a loss of bladder control. When young children are toilet-trained they learn bladder control by programming their brains to interrupt the natural reflex action of passing water without restraint. What they learn to consciously control are the sphincter at the neck of the bladder and the detrusor muscles in the bladder wall. In MS there can be demyelination of the nerves which transmit messages between the brain and the bladder muscles. One common effect of this demyelination is feeling the need to dash to the toilet again and again. It makes for a very tiresome lifestyle, forcing you never to stray far from a toilet. It is often worth warning friends and colleagues about it in a brief, factual but light-hearted way. This is the type of incontinence doctors refer to when they ask if you have any problems with frequency and urgency. The bladder nerves have become overactive and are telling the bladder to empty before it is properly full.

Urge incontinence is when the bladder empties almost as soon as the desire to pass urine is felt. The detrusor muscles in the bladder wall go into a spasm without warning and the bladder has to act. It just can't wait for you to give the go-ahead. *Reflex incontinence* is

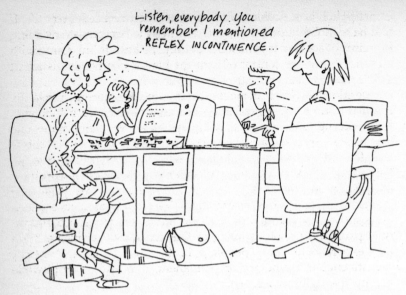

IT'S OFTEN WORTH WARNING YOUR FRIENDS AND COLLEAGUES ABOUT INCONTINENCE IN A BRIEF, FACTUAL AND LIGHT-HEARTED WAY..

similar only this time the message from the brain doesn't get through to check the reflex emptying of the bladder. This is what happens with bed-wetting.

Retention is the reverse problem – when you want to empty your bladder, you can't. It is prevented by a spasm or strong contraction of the sphincter. Sometimes the normal co-ordination between the sphincter and detrusor muscles goes awry. Urine is retained because the sphincter doesn't open properly and then is suddenly squeezed out because there are detrusor spasms in the bladder wall.

Bowel control

Losing control of the bowel leads to *faecal incontinence*. As this is generally caused by severe constipation, it is advisable to maintain bowel regularity or take steps to reestablish it if lost. A wholefood diet, rich in bran, wholemeal bread and pasta, brown rice and fresh fruit and vegetables provides the roughage needed to guard against constipation. It's also important to drink enough fluid and avoid too much refined food. If dietary changes do not do the trick then medical advice on which suppositories to use may be necessary.

Constipation is more common in people who live a sedentary life. If you have mobility problems, you may need to compensate by doing exercises of some sort to benefit not only the bowels but your health in general. Loss of control of both the bladder and bowel is called *double incontinence*.

Incontinence can become a severe problem during a relapse. Normal or much recovered improved control will return spontaneously during remission. It may always be an MS symptom or one that becomes more of a problem with age, but remember that this is true for the general population anyway. The person to go to for help initially is your GP who may refer you to a specialist or nurse continence advisor. The MS Society (for address see page 140) issues an excellent free information sheet on incontinence which gives more detailed information, and advice on drugs, catheterization, pads and various appliances that are widely available. With this expert help most people will be able to cope. Whether incontinence is temporary or permanent, it is always worthwhile getting the right advice.

Pain

'At least you don't get pain with MS' is one of those pieces of infuriatingly inaccurate information that too many people trot out as fact. When you reply that you do suffer pain your answer is largely dismissed. It is as if the person talking to you is saying that having MS is bad enough and pain in addition is too much. It is puzzling that for so long popular opinion, including the medical profession, has refused to believe that MS can be painful. Until recently, medical textbooks ignored the reality of pain in MS. Consequently even some neurologists have been surprised by the recent accumulation of evidence that many, but not all, people with MS experience pain. The pain spectrum runs from minor aches and pains common to most people through to MS revolving around pain. Pain relief clinics report that persistent pain in MS is one of the trickiest problems they have to deal with. The cause of pain is difficult to diagnose and to cure at the best of times and particularly so if MS is involved.

Pain is very real to the person who is suffering it and very frightening. It is taken as a sign that something is wrong, physically or emotionally. Pain is generally accepted as a serious warning to be taken notice of. However, as far as MS is concerned, pain does not indicate a worsening of the disease. It may have nothing to do with MS at all, and even if it does, it is a result of MS and not a sign of deterioration. The pain associated with MS can be the direct result of MS lesions and thus termed *neurological* in origin, or it can be *musculoskeletal*.

Neurological pain

The neurological types of pain (known as *parasthesias*) include pins and needles anywhere, tingling, shivering sensations, weird burning pains as if you were on fire, feelings of pressure and heightened sensitivity to touch on isolated tender patches of the skin or teeth. These pains cover the whole spectrum of aching, throbbing, stabbing, shooting, gnawing and tingling. In addition, peculiarly uncomfortable feelings of tightness and numbness are often reported. Any part of the body can be affected but most commonly it is the limbs, neck and head. Demyelination causes the brain to be misinformed about what is going on in the periphery of the body. There is defective conduction of nerve impulses. Much of the work of the central nervous system is to shut out distracting sensations in order to concentrate on carrying out everyday tasks. Interference with this results in being bombarded with sensations you don't want and can't control, including pain.

There are some common types of neurological pain in MS. *Trigeminal neuralgia* is thought to result from demyelination of the sensory nerve to the face. It is felt on the side of the head or face and is often triggered by, for example, cold or being touched. It is very unpleasant and depressing if it lasts long. The pain is usually relieved by taking Tegretol (Carbarnazepine). If this doesn't work, alcohol injections into the nerve may be effective. *Hermitt's parasthesia* is a sudden but brief pain down the back and into the legs and arms that occurs when bending the neck. It can vary in sensation from a sharp electric shock type pain to a tingling or pins and needles pain. The only way to cope with it is to avoid bending the neck. Wearing a collar support helps.

Optic neuritis is another unpleasant pain which affects the eyes. It is a sharp pain, like the cut of a knife, felt when moving one or both eyes. The eyeballs usually feel tender, and there is often an accompanying headache. It may also be associated with blurred vision which can last from moments to weeks. It probably results from the stretching of the meninges surrounding the swollen optic nerve. Optic neuritis is a common first symptom of MS. It usually lasts no more than a few days. If severe and longer lasting, this pain may be relieved by treatment with steroids.

Sometimes a continuous sciatica-like pain in one leg, part of the trunk or in an arm can set in and become very troublesome. This pain (*pseudoradicular*) varies in intensity and may be experienced as clammy coldness or a burning heat. The MS lesions responsible are probably located in the sensory tracks, or roots, of the spinal cord. It is difficult to treat because drugs, such as Tegretol that relieve the pain, usually have the side-effect of weakening the muscles and affecting the way you walk by causing the legs to cross in front of each other in a scissor-like movement.

Headaches aren't generally much different from normal when you have MS. Tension headaches can persist for weeks or months prior to the onset of MS, and probably result from physical or emotional stress. They can recur periodically for the same reasons. It is important that doctors check whether a headache has a cause other than demyelination and treat it accordingly.

Musculoskeletal pain

Musculoskeletal pain affects the muscles and bones and is most often experienced in the hips, tailbone, legs and arms. It usually arises when muscles, tendons and ligaments remain immobile for a while. The most severe and debilitating of these are muscular flexor spasms which result from demyelination in the spinal cord. They are most noticeable when they come just as you are dropping off to sleep or jolt you awake in the middle of the night. Your partner may also experience pain of a different sort if he or she is on the receiving end of a leg spasm.

Treating pain

Treating pain is difficult and each individual will need to experiment to find out the best method of relieving their particular pain. Doctors recommend trying drugs first before turning to less orthodox means of control, such as biofeedback or acupuncture. Generally speaking, if you suffer from muscle-type pain, you need to move about more and keep changing position. If you can't manage an exercise programme, try spending a few minutes in a rocking chair or get someone to gently move each limb in turn. Physiotherapy and/or massage are very beneficial. Check you are lying on the right sort of mattress for you, perhaps even try a water bed – the feel of warm water may cause the muscles to respond more easily to being moved.

If your pain is neurological in origin, you may find that in addition to painkillers, taking an antidepressant is helpful. This is because it modifies the way the central nervous system reacts to pain. Sensation pains often respond to the application of greater pressure, heat or cold.

If all else fails, a doctor can refer you to a specialist pain clinic. As part of the treatment, they will stress the emotional and psychological components of pain. Pain fast becomes the focus of all that is wrong in life. It is the strongest statement the body can make as it screams to be attended to. It gives you a legitimate reason to go to a doctor for help.

Living with pain

Pain affects you in many ways. It stops you being fully involved in life, often forcing you to withdraw from the company of others to suffer in isolation. It is depressing and can push some people towards thoughts of suicide. When you are putting up with pain, your thinking shuts down and you can't be bothered about life around you or concerned about the problems of others. Your senses are affected – being touched can be so sore, lights painfully bright and glaring, hearing loud, discordant and jumbled, heat exhausting and enervating, cold tooth-grinding and numbing, and damp bone-aching. Pain sets everything on edge.

Pain also allows you a voice. It gets attention and sympathy from those who see your distress. It allows you to avoid unpleasant situations and to get out of doing what you don't like. It gives you reasons to cover up your feelings or express them in an outburst. It gives you power to get people to do what you want.

Living with pain can persist when the physical reason for the pain has gone. Pain can become a way of life if you have tolerated it for a long time. That can be countered by finding ways of bringing back enjoyment, fun and laughter into life. Many people remark on the fact that they can forget their pain while they are doing something they enjoy or spending time with friends they like. Being cheerful and outgoing has a positive effect on the body, producing a kind of chemical reaction that deadens some pain. There is obviously some truth in the proverb that a merry heart does you as much good as medicine.

Fatigue

Have you ever started to tell someone just how unwell you were feeling only to be cut short by 'But you look so good!'? All the niggling symptoms you were noticing and wanted to share and the fact that you felt exhausted were brushed aside as apparently untrue. How can you look so good when you feel so rotten? It can take a while to register externally what your body is telling you loud and clear inside – that it is tired. By the time you look fatigued, you have usually gone far beyond your limits.

Fatigue can be a major MS symptom but one that is hard to verify objectively. It is relatively easy to see if someone has any paralysis or tremor, or to check eyesight problems. Fatigue affecting the function of the senses and muscles is not identifiable in the same way. It is an all-pervasive symptom, an integral part of MS and hard to understand.

Practically everyone knows what it's like to be tired and those who don't will never understand anyway. MS fatigue is more than ordinary tiredness. There is something natural about being healthily tired after a good day's work or a strenuous game of squash. That is not true about MS fatigue. You only realize the difference when it lifts and you are relieved of its debilitating effect. It can hit you suddenly and dramatically as if a plug was taken out and all your energy had drained away – you are zapped. Or it can creep up on you imperceptibly and you find yourself slowing down, dragging along with no push left. Everything is much more of an effort. Most of the time fatigue is tolerable – a gnawing unease and lack of bounce. At its worst it's like the worst type of 'flu without the cold symptoms and verging on a semiconscious state.

It is important to be aware of the differences between normal tiredness and fatigue. It is normal to be tired and ready to rest at the end of a day, when you have overworked, or not had enough sleep. MS fatigue happens faster, lingers longer and takes longer to recover from. One night's sleep will not always do the trick. It is not only a physical tiredness but a neurological one. The motor nerves are affected so that your muscles feel heavy and weak. You are likely to experience poor co-ordination, shakiness and exaggerated or inverted reflexes. The sensory nerves are affected too. Eyesight can become blurred, speech slurred, hearing and the sense of taste and smell dulled. The sense of touch can be impaired and accompanied by tingling or numbness. Vertigo can become troublesome.

Psychological factors

Psychological factors also play an intricate role in how you experience fatigue. Fatigue is bound to have a depressive effect and results in some anxiety. This is in addition to the anxiety and depression that frequently accompany MS anyway and are expressed in feelings of tiredness, lack of energy and heaviness. The effect is doubled.

It's difficult to assess from a clinical point of view what is actually fatigue, what is a reaction to MS and what is a depressive or anxiety state. It is no wonder that some people with MS fatigue are misdiagnosed as neurotic first. Doctors have some patients who hide or fail to identify the existence of fatigue as an MS symptom. They are in contrast to those who appear to over-react to fatigue and exaggerate their symptoms, often dramatizing them in an emotional way. So it is understandable that faced with such different reactions, doctors may not properly understand how real a symptom fatigue is.

Trigger factors

Fatigue is caused in two ways. The demyelinated nerve fibres use up more energy than normal as they conduct impulses. They tire quickly with use and the result is increased weakness and lack of co-ordination. It really does not take much to tire the central nervous system. The other reason for fatigue is that some muscles have to work extra hard to compensate for the weakened ones and so get tired faster. This is in addition to energy output being already reduced in MS and so normal muscle fatigue is felt more often and more quickly. This helps explain why you may look well, initially feel well, and start off doing something well only to then suddenly have to stop because of fatigue.

There seem to be some common trigger factors. Fatigue is often brought on by doing too much, infection, heat, smoking, drinking, overeating or by engaging in any activity for too long without a break. For example a rise in body temperature makes all the difference if your body is in a borderline state as is often the case with MS. Within a day it is normal for body temperature to fluctuate and reach a peak in the afternoon. It helps to find out what your low ebb times are so you do not plan anything demanding then. Pam regularly rests straight after lunch to get over her tired spot in the day and finds that gives her the energy to cope with the children when they get home from school. Also, people with MS may not always be aware that they are fighting infection. Samantha has noticed that she rarely comes down with the bugs that lay her colleagues off sick, but she often feels very tired at that time, presumably because her body is fighting off infection.

Whatever the trigger, MS fatigue appears like a psychological reaction rather than the physical one it really is. Fatigue does, however, have a pronounced effect on symptoms. It is as if there were a well of MS symptoms under the surface that only reach the top and show themselves when you are tired. You may feel you are heading for a relapse but these old symptoms only return temporarily. Also temporary is a common but slight personality change that can accompany fatigue. You feel out of step with yourself and under the weather.

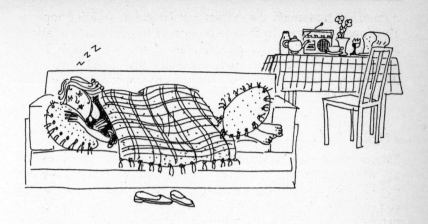

PAM REGULARLY RESTS STRAIGHT AFTER LUNCH TO GET OVER
HER TIRED SPOT IN THE DAY...

Working with fatigue

Fatigue is not harmful so long as you do not fight it but work round
it. Struggling to keep going at all costs is counterproductive. If you
become fatigued for a long period of time and do not get enough
sleep and rest, you run the risk of serious physical harm which
takes a long time to reverse. Sometimes you have to fight yourself
first before you rest as you know you need to. It's a fight against
pride when you need to be always in control and forcing the issue.

Life becomes easier by learning to recognize fatigue before it
catches up with you. What helps most is pacing and planning the
day with rest and relaxation periods built in. Burning the candle at
both ends just does not work with MS. It is best to simplify your
lifestyle and your home to your needs. It also helps to keep
physically fit, eat healthily and give up smoking. Being able to share
all this with someone who accepts the truth of MS helps so much. It
relieves a lot of tension, and feels very supportive.

Fatigue is becoming increasingly recognized as a serious symptom of MS by the medical profession. Other medical professionals
such as physiotherapists and occupational therapists also need to be
educated to take into account its pervasive effect. People with MS
may have to be firm about what they know they can and cannot do
on any given day because of fatigue and not allow themselves to be
bullied into doing more than they should. Family and friends also
need to have explained to them how necessary it is for those with
MS to conserve their energy to spend it on whatever they decide are
priorities.

'Twilight zones' of MS

These are transitory set-backs, slow-downs and low times. They are elusive experiences that are difficult to define. People with MS often talk about feelings and experiences to do with MS that are personal and subjective. They are not mentioned in texts on MS but deserve to be given an airing. For want of a better expression I choose to call them 'twilight zones'.

Experiencing a 'twilight'

The stark reality of these 'twilight zones' is that a lot is going on and not only on one level. It is easy enough to focus on physical symptoms, or emotional reactions, or psychological musings, or events, places, people, diets, allergies and the like, and to disregard the totality of the experience. All these factors are part of a complex interrelationship. This is when you can lose sight of who you are, although you may still have some control and are not being taken over completely. You still feel some vestige of yourself – that you are a real, whole person.

You may feel your energy is gone and you do not know where feelings begin and end and what pain is linked to what sensation. You doubt the provability of any particular symptom and wonder if you are somehow imagining the strange jumbling of sensations, thoughts and feelings. Now is the time to relax and accept that this is another of the faces of MS. It is a most misunderstood phase, disputed even by some doctors, family and friends. This is hardly surprising for those with MS have often spent hours of internal dialogue, disputing whether what is happening is real. To cope you must accept that it is very real. In practical terms, if you have MS you need to give yourself space and time to relax and soak up positive experiences. You need to rest as much as you want to and to do only what you want to do, as far as that is possible.

Rest and coping

What happens if you do not rest? You may indeed get away with it this time. You may by will-power and sheer determination, talk yourself out of it or through it, by putting yourself into 'overdrive'. Although you may succeed in pushing it out of mind and out of sight, it will have left its mark. Repeated setbacks similarly dealt with leave a series of marks that eventually have to be reckoned with.

When the crunch comes, a person is overtaken and suffers a severe relapse. All you can do is give in. It then takes a slower, uphill fight to get back on your feet. Now you are really in the invalid role again and it is obvious to everyone. The clear loss of energy and inability to manage everyday life indicate without doubt that you are sick.

Some cope by choosing this option. It buys what can be called 'legitimate space'. Everyone around has to admit that the person concerned has MS and is incapacitated by it. It is an unpopular way of coping, because everyone suffers. It is a source of disgruntlement and strains relationships. However, there was a time, during the 'twilight zone' experience that preceded the relapse, when a warning was given. There was a chance at that point to salvage something and take action to ease the situation. Maybe even the relapse itself could have been prevented. So much is learnt in retrospect. What is more challenging is to experiment in advance by accepting one's individual experiences of MS and taking care to act then.

Exacerbations

During an exacerbation there is an increase in pre-existing symptoms. This is most often brought on by infection or fever. Exposure to heat, trauma, stress and other metabolic changes may also trigger an exacerbation.

What it feels like

An exacerbation may last anything from a few minutes to a very long time. If an exacerbation comes suddenly, the person concerned will experience not only a recurrence of symptoms but also a shock to the system. Some say that they can feel fine one minute but the next they are aware of MS symptoms like a bolt from the blue. They cope with resilience at the time but may experience an emotional reaction later as they adjust to the shock factor.

At other times there is a gradual build-up to an exacerbation. During the build-up you have a problem accepting that you do not feel so well. Evidence is so subjective and you may experience times of confusion and conflict, when there is a gap between what you should do and feel and what you really can do and feel. Recent research into the common cold indicates that well before symptoms become apparent, the brain has already registered the start of the cold. It seems to be like that with MS too. During this build-up it is common to be highly emotional. Some people may cry a lot or feel unusually isolated from others and fearful that they are not acceptable.

Friends and relatives of people with MS need to understand that this is quite common and part of a normal reaction. What people experiencing this desperately want at this time is tangible acceptance, love and support. They need supersensitive reassurance and understanding of how raw they feel. They do not need jollying out of it, but appreciation that they are acutely distressed with an exacerbation and are probably unable to differentiate between what is meant and what is a joke. Their mental processes may slow down too.

During exacerbations people may consciously try to control their behaviour. It is a characteristic way of trying to restore stability in life when it has become rocky and unstable. If a person can make sure that something will happen in a certain way or that someone will do what they want, they feel in command of part of their life still.

Coping with exacerbations

It is essential to find out how to cope with exacerbations. On the practical level you should shield yourself from getting overtired. The body needs to conserve energy to fight the exacerbation. Rest when necessary but do not become immobile. The aim should be to move about a little and build this up gradually until a normal state of mobility is reached now and again. Gentle exercise and massage may be helpful. If the main symptom is excessive fatigue, a person may feel he or she will never again have the strength to do more than just lie prone. However, the body will recover its strength and, as it does so in slow stages, make sure that normal activity begins as soon as it can.

It makes good sense to cancel appointments and any engagements that might cause particular strain. It is also a good idea to refuse deadlines and not to tackle problems, especially relationship ones. It is remarkable how effective letting yourself off the hook is. When you let go of pressures, you often find you feel restored quite quickly. Mary, a student with MS, suffered an exacerbation as she was working on a thesis with a deadline to meet. She was forced to accept that she would not make the deadline, put aside her work for a few days and rested. Within 24 hours she felt her symptoms easing and was well enough to resume study. There is something healing about giving in to your body and being guided by what it says it needs during an exacerbation. It is a sort of pampering that is not indulgence but common sense.

During an exacerbation a person may struggle with feelings of neediness. You may be the sort who normally attends to the needs of others and puts your own needs in the background. It is important to resolve this and find out how best your needs can be met. Often you need to release your feelings. A good howl with a stock of tissues can work wonders. You may want to be alone or very close to others, taking comfort from support and physical closeness.

It is the person with MS who is the expert when it comes to dealing with his or her own exacerbations. It is individual experience that counts – there is no need for anyone else to validate it. Although an exacerbation is an integral part of MS, it is unnecessary to give it more weight than it deserves. It will not go on for very long and while it does you should try to feel positive about yourself, keeping your value as a person separate from the distorted experience of an exacerbation.

Sexual problems

Oliver is a good-looking virile young man whose MS was affecting his sex life. He needed to reach out, love and be loved in his marriage but the fact that he could not maintain an erection and suffered occasional impotence had put paid to any lovemaking as far as his wife was concerned. He just could not perform conventionally and his wife was not prepared to accept any other options sexually. They shut off from each other, stopped trying and stopped communicating their need for each other. He felt guilty because he was unable to satisfy his wife. They both needed each other sexually and it hurt badly when it seemed that that part of their relationship was over. As a result Oliver found himself attracted to someone at work and before long was involved in a secret love affair in which he and his new partner found and enjoyed alternative ways of making love.

Common problems

Oliver is an example of how a sexual problem can be allowed to go unresolved and cause detrimental separation between partners. It also illustrates the fact that there are always other options when it comes to expressing love. Unlike Oliver, you may never be affected sexually. For instance when it comes to sexual libido most people with MS experience a normal drive, a few experiencing an increased one. When MS does interfere with sexual activity it is inability or reduced ability in the physical expression of sex that is most apparent, although psychological factors are of equal importance. The sexual problems that result differ from person to person, vary between relapse and remission, and are affected by fatigue. The 'too tired tonight' line takes on extra significance with MS.

Men with MS may become impotent, find it difficult to get and maintain an erection and be aware of changes in the timing, nature and sensation of ejaculation. Women with MS may lack sensation as a result of the lack of clitoral engorgement, and may notice a lack of vaginal lubrication. Spasms in the thigh muscles may occur, making it difficult to have intercourse. For both men and women, it is usually necessary to try out new positions when there is muscular weakness, spasm or easy fatigue.

Finding solutions

The reasons for sexual problems may be neurological but they may also be emotional or a mixture of the two. It is certainly possible to get help with emotional problems and it is also possible to find alternative ways of expressing love sexually if the problem is a result of demyelination. Some doctors, counsellors and psychotherapists specialize in helping people with sexual problems. People make love for a host of good reasons and there is every reason to continue lovemaking even if MS tries to interfere. Sexuality is a vital part of a person's total personality. When you are satisfied sexually, you enjoy a completeness that pervades the whole of you. The reverse is also true. If there are problems and pressures in other parts of your life, your sex life feels the effect.

Even before diagnosis, it is quite likely that MS was affecting sexual activity. It may have caused fatigue or unexplained moodiness or direct loss of sexual function. That will have placed a strain on sexual relationships. Once people know they have MS, they may fear that sexual activity will make their condition worse, though this is in fact highly unlikely unless a person allows himself or herself to become overtired. A little discreet forward planning can normally overcome that problem.

To cope well sexually, you need to consider first your definition of what sexual activity is. If you insist on narrowly defining it as the ability to have sexual intercourse conventionally, you are limiting your sexual expression and satisfaction. It is legitimate to discover there really is no right way, and no need for 'shoulds' in a good loving sexual relationship. On the other hand there is plenty of room for discovering new ways of relating.

You also need to become aware of the problems anyone can have in a sexual relationship and then consider the added problems of MS. Any man with impotence experiences frustration and tends to avoid intercourse because he is afraid of repeated failure. If MS is likely to be the cause and it threatens to be so permanently, then the man's confidence will be knocked twice over. Similarly a woman may avoid intercourse because she can't enjoy it in the way she used to and she feels she has failed too, even if there is MS to blame.

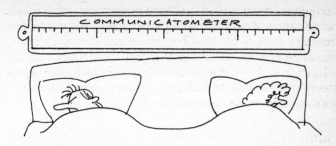

... SEX EASILY BECOMES THE SCAPEGOAT FOR ANY SHAKY MARRIAGE. IT IS A SORT OF BAROMETER, REGISTERING ADVERSELY ANY BREAKDOWN IN COMMUNICATION ...

Both have lost a means of expressing love sexually and spontaneously, a loss that needs to be grieved about before new approaches can be found.

It is also a common experience for those who feel unattractive, for whatever reason, to believe they are unlovable and do not warrant sexual relations. If they are also struggling to accept their MS and whatever disability, visible or invisible that goes with it, they may find that they distance themselves from a sexual partner and ignore or negate the love offered. Or the reverse may be true. They may so crave reassurance that they are still lovable, that they make unacceptable demands to try and compensate for the negative feelings they have about themselves.

Sex easily becomes the scapegoat for any shaky marriage. It is a sort of barometer, registering adversely any breakdown in communication and closeness. It is sensitive to unexpressed feelings, especially a backlog of anger. If the physical effects of MS on sexual function are not taken into account, there is plenty of scope for misunderstanding. Unresolved sexual problems can become reason enough for your relationship to flounder.

It is easy to fear that a partner will seek sexual satisfaction elsewhere. In the main such fears are unfounded. Strong feelings of jealousy may be more strongly felt, partly as the result of the effect MS can have on the emotions. There may be, after all, many more opportunities for a partner to make new relationships, but frequently that partner feels as much jealousy when the partner with MS has to be cared for by nursing staff at home or in hospital.

If someone becomes disabled to the degree where he or she needs help with washing, feeding and toileting, and a partner takes this on for them, there may be a change of emphasis in the relationship. There is a potential role conflict when a partner becomes more of a nurse than a lover. Physical contact can easily become limited to the basic essentials of nursing care. There may actually be a need to confront this by specifically encouraging affectionate warm sexual contact. If it is finally decided to discontinue a sexual relationship, this decision should always be reached mutually and not by default.

There are three basic needs to fulfil if you want a good sexual relationship. The first is to communicate well. This involves expressing your feelings and being willing to talk frankly and without embarrassment. It helps to share specifically what you like and dislike sexually, what you expect in the relationship and what approaches to sexual activity you are willing to take.

The second need is for intimacy. You deserve to keep a deep and intimate closeness. If one partner has MS this may involve finding new ways of being close which at first may feel inadequate, but which are certainly worth investing in. If intercourse is either impossible or ill-advised, caressing, stroking and long warm hugs help maintain sexual closeness. It is also best to continue to sleep in the same bed. If MS leads to a period in hospital or long-term care away from home, special arrangements may have to be made to keep intimate times going.

The third need is to explore. People with MS may have to make the best of a bad situation and initially feel too unnatural and frightened to try new approaches. But if they really want to give pleasure as well as to receive it, it is important to seek information on alternative ways of making love, making use of different techniques, sexual aids and more comfortable positions. It is also important to know how to cope with incontinence problems and catheters, and maintain careful personal hygiene. There are excellent books on the market, some written for the general public and others specifically to cover sex and disability. Several organizations also exist to give advice and help in this area (for addresses, see page 140). You may also consider seeing a counsellor who specializes in helping couples with sexual problems.

Meeting psychological barriers

The greatest psychological struggle people with MS have to face is to do with fear and prejudice. This includes both their own fear and prejudice and that of others. This confrontation occurs firstly at diagnosis and then on and off afterwards, if ever or whenever the symptoms of MS prove disabling in any way. To be aware of this situation helps. To be able to give it a name and to recognize it for what it is limits its power. A person can then choose what weight to give it in his or her life.

Fear

Even if MS remains invisible, those who have it will never be entirely free of occasional niggling fears. They are those momentary 'what if' fears that should be acknowledged, but should then be dismissed. Chances are that if ever these fears do become reality, the strength to cope will then be found somehow. That is also true for fears more firmly based on fact. Accept that they may be valid at some future point in time, but that for now they can be forgotten.

There are times when fears build into a panic. Many factors can be involved in this – personality type, experience of life, relationships, the situation at home, work, general state of health, and, not least, the fact of living with a neurological disease affecting the central nervous system. Panic is temporary – it will pass. There is no need to do anything about it except to give it time to release itself and settle.

Prejudice

There is a very real but unspoken prejudice against disability and whatever indicates the presence of disability. It may be a prejudice you are already aware of in yourself or others. It can even be a prejudice that people with MS feel towards themselves. While it is more common to experience this prejudice in the face of visible disablement, it is also possible to experience it when facing the effects of invisible symptoms.

The prejudice against disability is obvious in people who grumble about those in wheelchairs cluttering up the pavement or shops and who are impatient to get past someone walking slowly with a stick. What is happening to people with the prejudice is that the aids – wheelchair or stick – get in the way and obscure the personality of the individual using them. They focus on what frightens and threatens them and are unable to take a broader view. The more severe the disability, the greater the threat.

MS with its fluctuating pattern and periods of deterioration during relapse poses a threat. Those who have to confront MS are placed in a quandary as they consider how severe their disability is, what its long-term effect could possibly be, and how predictable and controllable its outcome. The conclusions drawn may determine whether or not help is offered and acceptance given. If neither is readily on offer, the person with MS will feel rejected and isolated.

It is a fact that certain illnesses carry more of a stigma than others. Heart attacks do not appear to have the stigma that MS does. The causes, treatments and prevention of heart attacks are understood and clear-cut in a way that MS is not. Frequently people with MS, their families and friends show they are in a way ashamed of the disease and its symptoms. The mystery of what causes it and the unpredictability of its course make them defensive. This defensiveness is put down to MS, but is more to do with the stigma of the disease. MS has a bad press – it is feared and is threatening. The stigma of MS is something else to grapple with and resolve, but you should never take on the responsibility for the effect of MS upon others. You may be able to make them aware of it and you may have to learn to accept that you can do nothing to change other people's reactions. Some people will avoid contact with anyone with MS and feel guilty about it. They are struggling with their own inability to overcome prejudice against a disabling illness. It can be more disabling for them to cope with the stigma than for the person with MS to cope with the disease. They find themselves watching carefully to make sure they say the 'right' things and to not let it be obvious that they are finding the situation difficult. They emphasize the positive at all times because they are afraid to feel and express any negative emotions especially anger towards someone with MS, in case the prejudice slips out and is revealed. It must be stressed that this is rarely a prejudice that anyone admits to. It seldom surfaces at a conscious level. It is not calculated in any way. It is an unconscious fear with far-reaching effects on relationships.

This section has focused on the way that MS can limit and change social relationships. People with MS need to be aware of the fact that MS can disable not only them, but in a different but very real way it can also disable their families, friends and others they come across. The family, in particular, runs the risk of being most seriously affected by prejudice against disability and may also experience the effects of stigmatization. It happens most easily when MS is handled as something fragile that they are afraid to talk about normally and dare not laugh about. They get into a pattern of allowing MS too important a place in their lives. It is people themselves that count and the practicalities of coping with disability should not intrude or predominate. Sadly, however, MS at its rare worst does demand a high degree of physical care and attention, placing a heavy burden on those who do the caring. If this happens, support of a special kind can minimize the intrusion of MS and it is still possible to maintain warmth and openness in relationships. This will be discussed in the pages that follow.

Impaired mobility

At some time or other people with MS are likely to experience difficulty in using their legs and arms. This is a crisis because of the dramatic effect loss of mobility has on the body and consequently on lifestyle generally. Not being able to walk well or use your arms normally feels wrong and is alarming to others. Obviously there must be something wrong when, for example, you find it increasingly difficult to walk, moving firstly from using a stick to a frame, and then needing a wheelchair for trips outside the house and finally for permanent use inside as well. Prolonged loss of mobility is generally associated with the progressive stages of MS. What is not known is how temporary mobility problems will be and how much they are going to interfere with life. It works well to assume they are not going to last and at the same time make use of whatever help is needed to get around easily. Edith needed to use a stick and then a wheelchair more or less permanently for some years. Today, however, she walks normally and has taken up cycling again. Some time ago she wrote to cancel the mobility allowance she had been granted for the rest of her working life because her walking problems had been so severe. She no longer needed it. Impaired mobility may not actually reflect any deterioration in someone's MS, but is rather a sign of where a lesion is located and evidence of a relapse.

Balance and co-ordination

Mobility is affected by a number of different factors, which include problems of balance and co-ordination, tremor and spasticity. It is helpful to be aware of what can hinder smooth spontaneous movement.

Poor or lost balance, often referred to as *vertigo*, has a devastating effect on the way someone normally gets around. It can be fleeting or last for several weeks. It is a sort of dizziness in which the pavement can seem to pitch, roll and toss like a boat-deck in a storm. Some people also feel nauseous, and may even get to the point of vomiting. Trying to walk with this going on is distressing and energy-consuming. Also, it is not always obvious to other people why someone is experiencing difficulty. A stick can be useful to give balance and warn others. Vertigo is normally accompanied by weakness and fatigue as well. Even when not trying to move about, vertigo can still persist. If very severe, even

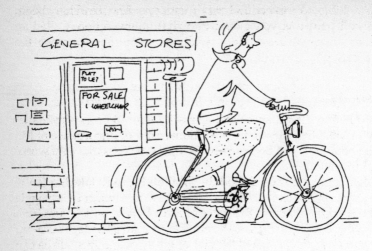

EDITH NEEDED TO USE A STICK, THEN A WHEELCHAIR MORE OR LESS PERMANENTLY FOR SOME YEARS. TODAY, HOWEVER, SHE WALKS NORMALLY AND HAS TAKEN UP CYCLING AGAIN...

lying flat and not moving at all does not take it away. In such cases all that can be done is to rest and see if any type of medication helps. Fortunately, vertigo is usually only mildly bothersome and clears up quite quickly.

Lack of normal co-ordination of the legs, arms or both has a clear affect on the ability to move normally. At times it can become a source of embarrassment for poorly co-ordinated legs produce a staggering gait that any drunkard would be proud of. It is a gait known as *ataxia* and has been described as a scissors walk. It was the sort of walking problem Kate was struggling with, her legs crossing in front of each other going their own wilful way. It was important to her that she saw her young daughter to and from school each day but hard to manage. She had so far hidden her diagnosis from her neighbours and the other mothers at the school gate, but she could not hide the evidence of her MS walk. Only when she learned that people thought she had taken to drink did she decide to share the fact that she actually had MS. She was warmed by the support and genuine concern she received. Practical help came her way as others offered to share in fetching her daughter from school when necessary.

Sometimes it is arms rather than legs that are affected. You reach out to take or return something and miss. This can be expensive in terms of broken crockery and very frustrating. The hand may begin to shake as soon as you intend to carry out any action. Called an *intention tremor*, this symptom results from interference along the nerve pathway.

Spasticity

Co-ordination disturbances and spasticity tend to occur simultaneously in MS. Spasticity is the predominant motor disturbance of MS and sometimes it can become severe. It is a stiffness that gets worse with movement.

Gillian knows that on a good day her stiff legs will take her to the local shops and back with the help of a stick. It is worth the struggle for the friendly chat and the sense of achievement on arriving back home with a few purchases. On not so good days her legs seize up by the time she has reached the end of her road and it is all she can do to get back to the house.

Spasticity is fatiguing and disabling and it is not worth forcing the body to achieve what it refuses to do. Instead let it ease up and coax it back into movement when it is ready. The drugs that are very effective against spasticity also have the side-effects of increasing weakness, so that the legs seem to turn to rubber. The medication enables suppleness to return to the limbs but they lose their strength to support. The one advantage of a spastic leg is that it can be used as a prop and pivot.

Spasms

Two particular types of spasm can become troublesome with MS and interfere with movement. *Extensor spasms* can occur when attempting to make a movement. Both legs shoot out straight and are then difficult or impossible to bend. It looks and feels alarming but is seldom painful. Sometimes bending the neck so the chin moves towards the chest can terminate the spasm. Extensor spasms often seem to occur at night, and rudely awaken you – and your partner.

Flexor spasms are usually a later development and are most often experienced by those in a chronic progressive stage of MS. The muscles involved here are those that bend the leg at the knee and hip joints. If you are on your feet at the time, the result of a flexor spasm is that you fall over. They are more painful and can happen when you are sitting or lying down too. Any infection of the bladder or any sore place on the legs seem to aggravate them. The drug Lioresal is of particular use as it acts specifically to dampen down any abnormally active reflexes. In the case of severe disability, more permanent measures like nerve-end blocking or surgical procedures may be needed, so you can sit or lie in comfort. The great fear with impaired mobility is always that it marks the start of a progressive stage that will catapult the sufferer into irreversible disablement. Such stages are characterized by a progressive decline in neurological function over a period of more than six months. They are rare early on, but more likely to develop after several years of MS. It seems that the prognosis is most favourable if MS follows a benign course for the first ten years.

When walking fails

Whenever MS affects mobility, it is time to consider alternative means of getting about. Not being able to rely on your own two legs to get you around is reason to panic. Sylvia recalls the time when the truth of her limited ability to walk really hit her hard. She was just beginning to feel that she was walking more steadily and picking up speed when one day a little old lady, clearly walking slowly and with some difficulty herself, not only caught her up but overtook her and disappeared round the corner. She felt devastated and sobbed when she got home. It just wasn't fair. For Sylvia it was a true crisis situation and she had to think long and hard about resolving it.

When it comes to mobility or lack of it, the choice is limited – discover new ways of staying mobile, remain confined and isolated at home, or depend on others. The first option is preferable in theory but in practice it is a tough option to follow. There are obvious reasons why people would rather not use a stick, a walking frame or a wheelchair. These are the badges of disability they would rather avoid. Society expects you to be either able-bodied or disabled and ignores the reality of a middle-ground. This needs confronting because life is full of experiences never faced before, that each individual must be helped to cope with. A wheelchair enables someone who cannot walk to stay mobile. A stick enables you to keep your balance. Using an orange badge enables you to park your car near the shops. Knowing when to make use of a stick or a wheelchair is difficult and is another of the potential crises of MS.

Take the prospect of using a wheelchair. It may so petrify you that you would rather stagger yourself to a standstill and collapse in a heap first. You may even be encouraged by doctors to keep out of a wheelchair as long as possible. They have a point because certainly there will always be a minority who use a wheelchair

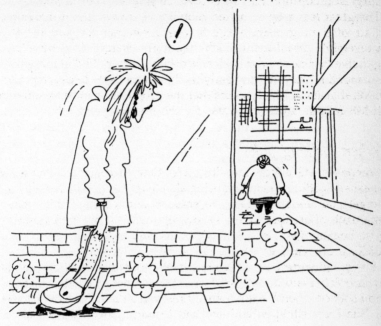

... A LITTLE OLD LADY, CLEARLY WALKING SLOWLY AND WITH SOME DIFFICULTY HERSELF, NOT ONLY CAUGHT HER UP BUT OVERTOOK HER AND DISAPPEARED ROUND THE CORNER ....

before they really need one. It is also conceivably a way to achieve the easy life or a sign that they have given up the fight. If such people lack power and ease in their lives to the extent that sitting in a wheelchair is going to resolve it, they need counselling help. Telling them to use a wheelchair as a last resort is not offering help where it is needed. Most people with MS need to be encouraged to use a wheelchair the way they use sunglasses – when the conditions really demand it. Using a wheelchair when it is absolutely necessary conserves energy and combats fatigue. Few parents would insist that their toddler, having once learnt to walk a few steps, should never again jump back into his pushchair. It makes sense to him and his parents to do so when he's tired or they need to get somewhere in a hurry.

Wheelchairs come in a more attractive range of colours, styles and size these days. They are either electrically-powered or manual, propelled by hand by the person in the wheelchair or pushed by someone else. It is less easy to be independent when you rely on another person to do the pushing. However, you need to have some strength and flexibility in your hands to control an electric wheelchair. It is usually worth persevering with one though, for the thrill of independence you get from being able to get around on your own. Scooters are an even more attractive alternative, as they are easily manoeuvrable and create a stir with the kids who hang around hoping you will get off and give them a go. Battery cars, are popular too, as they can be driven on the road and will travel many miles before they need recharging. The more people with MS and other disabilities make use of and have fun with their wheelchairs, scooters and the like, the sooner other people will be forced to change their preconceptions. Sitting in a wheelchair does not actually change you into a moron and it is high time that that misconception was challenged.

If mobility problems are to do with balance and co-ordination rather than spasticity, a stick or some other type of support may be enough. If you have young children, you will find a pram or pushchair useful to lean on. Shopping trolleys of the right kind can be a walking aid too. A walking frame may be useful – some have wheels attached and a basket or resting seat attachments.

Without doubt a car is the most convenient way to keep mobile where longer distances are involved. You may find it better to drive an automatic car or have controls adapted. It is easy to have hand controls fitted, and pedals can be adapted for left-foot acceleration in an automatic car too. If you are unable to walk or walk only with great difficulty, you may qualify for the Mobility Component of the Disability Living Allowance. There is also a Motability scheme which helps you use your Mobility Allowance to purchase and run a car. The orange badge scheme is invaluable because it allows the use of parking spaces designated for the disabled and gives the right to park for a limited time where no other vehicles can. The local offices of the Department of Health and Social Security will be able to provide you with details of these schemes.

Using public transport becomes virtually impossible when you have a problem walking and keeping your balance. You have to be somewhat agile to enter or leave a bus or railway carriage. If you have a disability that does not show, then it is worth carrying a stick to make it obvious, otherwise you can get jerked off your feet because the driver does not realize he should give you time to sit down first. Coach operators and British Rail are very obliging and make special provision if you have a mobility problem. You need to warn them in advance so they have time to make arrangements. The same is true when travelling by air. If you contact the airline ahead of time, they will make sure you and any escort get into your seats with a minimum of difficulty.

Long-term care

There will be times when there is a need to reflect on the meaning of life and death in the light of one's own vulnerability. It is normal and healthy to do so and having MS is a good enough reason to take stock. Some prefer to ponder on their own, while others want to work out ideas with the help of someone else. Often it is easier to do so with someone understanding, who has a distance from your immediate family and closest friends. It will help you to voice what is going on inside you and gives you courage as you consider the changes you would like to initiate in order to meet the future. At some stage it is wise to try and involve those close to you in discussing your future, providing you and they can cope with it.

Planning ahead

No one knows what lies ahead, but it makes good sense to begin to build into relationships what is needed to survive any eventuality. In practical terms this may mean arranging that people with MS and those caring for them can have time apart. People need a break and time for themselves. Although this is especially important if the person with MS becomes severely disabled, it is valid for anyone at any stage. There is a very real danger of being stifled in a claustrophobic relationship when people are together for 24 hours a day and 365 days a year. Similarly it is wise for people with MS to learn to accept physical care and attention from others. But if at all possible, try to make sure that one person does not have sole responsibility for washing, feeding or toileting.

Finding help

Others.– a district nurse or a home help for example – are usually available to come in and take on responsibility for routine physical care. Suitable nursing staff may be paid for under the conditions of some private medical insurance schemes. There is also the Crossroads Care attendance scheme (see page 143), a network of carers throughout the country who contract to come in and relieve on a regular basis. Using such outside help allows some space between people who need to be cared for and their family or friends who normally do the caring. It is unrealistic to expect from any single relationship everything you want at any time and on demand, even if you are related by blood or marriage. Yvonne came back home to live when she needed some looking after. However, she had never had an easy relationship with her mother and although they both tried hard, in the end they had to admit that Yvonne would be better off in a hostel catering for the disabled, where she did not need to be dependent on her mother but could still welcome occasional visits.

Day-to-day strain

There is no denying the strain involved in living day in and day out with disability, especially when you are largely physically dependent on others. It's too easy to become confined to four walls and find yourself and those caring for you becoming isolated from the mainstream of life. There is distress whenever you grapple with a slow slide towards any sort of incapacity, relief at any halting and joy when, despite all indications to the contrary, remission takes place. Dealing with practicalities can eat up so many hours and so much energy that it is difficult to hold on to some of the trimmings, so that life has quality and is not just a matter of existence. Twice a week Olga went back to her old school where she had been a teacher. There she spent a couple of hours listening to the children read and helping them with any reading problems. They loved the attention, found her wheelchair a novelty, and never minded that she could not move her arms and legs or talked in a funny way. She knew she was fulfilling a useful function.

Residential care

There may come a time when long-term residential care needs to be considered. This is usually an emotionally charged decision to make and for so many people it seems like an admission of failure. It is not easy for a partner or family to have to admit for whatever reason they cannot manage to continue to care for someone at home. Residential care in a private, local authority, health authority or voluntary-run home is an option that makes good sense when someone needs constant personal nursing care. It is an option that should be considered when the possibilities of additional help from district nurses or care assistants coming to the home on a daily basis have been exhausted. Remember though that although people may understand that they need special nursing care that perhaps only a residential home can give, they will not normally want to move from an intimate, family-type situation to being part of a large, less personal group. They will fear isolation and wonder whether their family and friends will remember to come and visit them after a while.

It is a fact that some families squeeze out a member with MS and are glad of the chance of residential care, but the reverse can also happen. Relationships previously under strain because of all the sheer hard physical work and long hours can and do improve dramatically. Visits become a pleasure and people enjoy a renewed relaxed warmth with each other.

Death

One of the taboo subjects in our society is death. Even talking about it is avoided. The only certainty after birth, it is best faced with calmness and dignity. If you have MS, you cannot help but die with it. Your MS may have nothing at all to do with your dying or it may be a contributory factor. Whichever is the case, it is wise to ensure that all personal affairs are in order and that, as far as possible, you are at peace with yourself and with others.

5

What help is on offer

Someone with a chronic disease like MS is bound to be smothered with concern and contradictory advice. Some of the treatments and sources of help outlined here may work but none is likely to be responsible for a 'cure' because it would be difficult to provide objective proof of one.

Scientific clinical trials are regularly carried out to investigate the

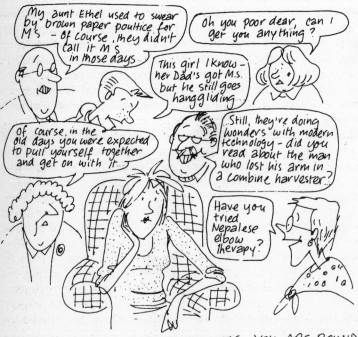

WITH A CHRONIC DISEASE LIKE MS YOU ARE BOUND TO BE SMOTHERED WITH CONCERN AND CONTRADICTORY ADVICE.

claims of certain treatments. These are normally part of a research project and are carried out with volunteer patients in hospital or an out-patients department. Inevitably, being involved in a clinical trial raises hopes and many choose to be part of such an experiment as a chance for treatment they would otherwise not get at that time. This is the case for trials on expensive drugs like beta-interferon. The fairness and equity about where trials are held, which people with MS are included, and how well prepared they are for the experience and outcomes are issues being addressed by MS societies and researchers, medical as well as pharmaceutical. Being involved in a clinical trial can become burdensome for several reasons: how frequent the visits have to be, the distance to be travelled, the wait for reimbursement, and, of course, the effects of the treatment under investigation.

Experimental treatment can be put to the test in one of three ways. In an open trial both the patients and doctors know what treatment is being tested and there is nothing to guard against subjective interpretation. It is a well-known fact that whatever treatment is administered, some people will inevitably feel better for it, at least for a while. In a blind controlled trial, only the doctor knows which patients are receiving the treatment under investigation and which are not. Thus the placebo effect is controlled but there is no control over the doctor's assessment, which may unconsciously bias the result. The only type of trial that receives full scientific acceptance is the double-blind controlled one.

The concept of the double-blind controlled trial is important. Neither the patients receiving the treatment nor those giving it know who is getting the actual drug, diet or whatever is being tested. Two groups of patients are needed and are carefully matched for age, sex and background. One group receives the treatment under investigation while the other – the control group – only appears to receive the same thing. The control group in fact gets something that either has no effect or one that has already been anticipated. Reactions to the treatment are carefully monitored. When the experiment is over, the identity of the groups is made known and results are analysed and assessed.

There is a world of difference between clinical testing under medical supervision and other treatments posing as cures. Only the patient can decide whether he or she wishes to try fringe treatments or alternatives to conventional medicine. There are many experimental therapies and treatments available. Many are offered by genuine, caring people who believe the evidence of their eyes, which is that some who underwent their special treatment got better. Satisfied customers are happy to testify to dramatic improvements in their condition, and this encourages others to try it.

Everyone wants to get better and this might do the trick. The danger is that you might be chasing the end of the rainbow, for a while at least, until disillusionment, a relapse or lack of energy, effort or finance put a stop to seeking a cure.

It is worth noting that people with MS and those who care for them will become most desperate to try and find a cure during a relapse. Yet it is just as likely at this time as at any other that spontaneous recovery will occur. Alternative treatments for MS abound and are added to regularly, some appearing to show benefit. Unless the proposed treatment undergoes double-blind controlled testing, it cannot be recommended. Even if no treatment at all is given, improvement is sure to come in a quarter of cases. If it comes while undergoing new treatment, its success will be attributed to that treatment, without any real justification.

Taking it all with a pinch of salt

What you believe in and fancy is sure to do you far more good than what you are sceptical about. Reading through this chapter, you are likely to dismiss some treatments as quackery, others as possible and a few as essential. Each has been included because at some time it has been linked with MS. None is a cure or a generally accepted treatment for MS but each has its devotees. It is up to individuals to decide what they want to try. It is likely that at some time and for some people, each may be just the job. It is worth experimenting, provided you remember a few safeguards. People with MS should never push themselves to exhaustion-point, physically, mentally or emotionally. Any therapy or treatment works best when you are relaxed and accepting. Any natural remedy takes longer to work than drugs and at first there may not be any positive indication that it is making any difference at all. People should only get involved with what they think will suit them personally and in terms of time, energy and money.

Drugs

From the 1950s on *corticosteroids* have been used to reduce the time of an MS relapse. The way they work is as blanket immunosuppressants, forcing the immune system to 'shut up and behave', so to speak. It is a definite relief to the person enduring an attack to have it curtailed in any way, even if there is only a short-term effect on disability along with some side-effects. So corticosteroids and other general immunosuppressive drugs continue to have an effective role in the treatment of MS and are offered in order to speed recovery from relapses. They have no long-term effect on overall disability. ACTH, probably the most popular of these, causes the adrenal glands to release steroids, and the most dramatic effect of any steroid treatment is the reduction of inflammation, a natural response of the body to injury. Both ACTH injections and intravenous methylprednisolone are equally effective in speeding up the rate of recovery from acute relapse. However, the latter seems to have fewer side-effects and may possibly have an additional effect on spasticity. Treatment with steroids can be given up to three or four times a year. Some describe this type of approach as heavy-handed, rather like using a sledge-hammer to tap in a tin-tack. However, similar treatments in combination with cyclophospha-mide or cyclosporine are more promising variations.

Until recently the only other drugs available apart from ACTH and corticosteroids were prescribed specifically to relieve the pain, spasticity, vertigo and incontinence that can occur with MS. Now at last there are new drugs – *beta-interferon-1a* and *1b* and copolymer-1 – that may noticeably affect the course of MS in a positive way. These are the first promising substances likely to have a measurable effect on the disease processes of MS itself rather than simply affecting the symptoms.

Interferons – alpha, beta and gamma – occur naturally in the body. They are chemical substances that act as messengers and play an important role in controlling the stimulation and suppression of the immune system. Some beta-interferons – beta-interferon-1b and 1a – are thought to be useful in MS because of their anti-viral response and the way they seem able to modulate the body's immune response. Currently there are different forms of beta-interferon on the market, each a marginally different chemical composition, administered by injection on a long-term basis. The brand names of these genetically engineered proteins are *Betaferon, Betaseron* and *Beneseron* (beta-interferon-1b), *Avonex* and *Rebif* (beta-interferon-1a), all of them working in a similar way.

The positive effect of beta-interferons is apparently to stop damage to the central nervous system by modifying some of the body's immunological pathways. This is the first drug to have a modulating effect on the underlying course of relapsing-remitting MS. Those with a mild form of this type of MS who take high doses of beta-interferon-1b can hope to experience up to one third fewer relapses. From MRI scans there is also evidence that lesion formation is reduced, but with no significant effect on disability. Reports on beta-interferon-1a which has been tested on people with relapsing-remitting and secondary progressive forms of MS, indi-cate a similar reduction in the relapse rate and lesion formation, and in addition fewer multiple relapses and an improvement in disability. Clearly beta-interferons are not a cure but an encouraging step forward. They certainly do not suit everybody.

The short-term side-effects of beta-interferon-1b, such as inflammation at the injection site and 'flu-like reactions, tend to pass, although there are reports of a depressive reaction, which for some people with MS can be intolerably severe. The side-effects of beta-interferon-1a are reported to be like a mild 'flu and mild anaemia. Any possible long-term side-effects are as yet unknown.

The major drawback to having beta-interferon prescribed is its very high cost. In addition, the fact that different forms of beta-interferon suit different types of MS must be borne in mind. Since the licensing of beta-interferon-1b in the United Kingdom, MS charities have been lobbying for this expensive drug to be made available in an equitable way to all who meet the clinical criteria, regardless of where they live.

Copolymer-1 (Copaxone) is another new drug that appears likely to modify the course of MS. It is not yet licensed for prescription but in clinical trials has been shown to have beneficial effects on people with relapsing and remitting MS. A complex of four amino acids, copolymer-1 is administered by daily self-injection. The clinical results seem to indicate a significant reduction in the relapse rate as well as an improvement in disability. The side-effects of copolymer-1 are reported to be minimal – some people have reactions at the site of the injections and a few experience a tight chest and shortness of breath.

Homoeopathy

Homoeopathy works on the principle that like cures like. It is an ancient method of healing, in which minute doses of a substance are prescribed. The substance chosen would produce the very symptoms you want to be rid of if it were given in larger doses. Homoeopathic medicines can be animal, vegetable or mineral in origin and are so dilute it is hardly credible that there is any potency left. Despite that, results are good but often slow. As these medicines work in animals as well as humans, their positive effects are more than just auto-suggestion.

Homoeopathy does not claim to cure MS but may provide specific remedies for certain of its symptoms, such as pain.

Herbalism

Herbal medicines are obtained solely from plants and contain no added chemicals. Herbalism was the main system of healing, an everyday part of life based on treating the whole person, from

Biblical times until early in the twentieth century. People with MS may find certain herbal treatments helpful. Herbal practitioners vary in the way they diagnose and carry out consultations. Check that a herbalist is registered, clean, consistent and honest. Natural remedies tend to take a longer time to work. Herbal treatments will never cure MS, but may alleviate symptoms and promote better health in general.

Cannabis

Some people with MS are reported to have found considerable benefit from using cannabis – they experience relief from distressing symptoms such as muscle spasm, especially in the bladder, tremors and pain. Others find no positive effect at all and a few have had negative reactions to cannabis, for example, impaired posture and balance.

As it is still illegal to prescribe cannabis, those with MS in favour of using it therapeutically are urging for a change in the law. They argue that cannabis is safe and non-addictive, despite the fact that it is a pharmacologically 'dirty' drug, containing a host of ingredients and actions, which are promising as well as problematic. The initial surveys highlighting the positive use of cannabis for MS need to be followed by full clinical trials to establish which active components in this complex organic compound are beneficial, neutral or harmful. Meanwhile some find the synthetic cannabinoid nabilone, which can be prescribed, gives reasonably good results.

Individually initiated drug treatment

When you have MS it is wonderful to find yourself suddenly free of the symptoms and on your feet again – literally. It is as if you have been given your life back again with the added bonus of wisdom and experience, gained at a price from juggling your life with MS. This sort of release comes spontaneously and the inevitable question is 'Why?'

Although many people with MS have rejoiced at dramatic improvements in their condition, it has taken someone with determination and foresight like Cari Loder to publish her own experience of 'recovery' and initiate a possible treatment for others. Cari Loder's therapeutic drug treatments (a combination of an antidepressant, amino acid and vitamin B_{12}) claims to compensate for the effects of nerve damage caused by MS and other demyelinating conditions. What has worked well for her and for some others in a self-selected group of volunteers is to undergo a full clinical trial, the results of which it is hoped will give confirmation of its efficacy.

Physiotherapy

Physiotherapy has been called the cornerstone of treatment for MS and is beneficial at all its stages. It is a programme of exercises designed to prevent or relieve any movement disorders, to ease mobility and to reduce the possibility of deformity.

The skill of the physiotherapist is to use exercises tailored specifically to individual needs. Physiotherapy will work well if the patient is motivated to keep the exercises up regularly, with a balance of effort and relaxation. The aim of physiotherapy is to maintain mobility and suppleness, so that the patient is able to be self-reliant and carry out the functions of everyday living.

It is important to become aware of the range of help physiotherapy can give. For example it is all too easy to slip into walking with a twisted posture or awkward gait as an unconscious compensation for a stiff leg or balance problem. The physiotherapist knows how to systematically exercise limbs and muscles, correct poor posture, improve muscle tone and work towards improved control of movement. Certain exercises help to restore balance and co-ordination. If fatigue is a problem, it may be that short periods of exercise sandwiched between rest periods can help to increase stamina and endurance. Its benefits are not only physical but psychological too. It helps with MS to have support from someone who is concerned with and understands the difficulties MS brings. Physiotherapists also have a good reputation among health-care professionals for their counselling approach.

One way of combating spasticity and co-ordination problems is to begin physiotherapy early on when problems may only be minor. Initially an intensive training programme of exercises is needed. It must be matched to individual needs and aimed at maintaining general mobility. The right exercises will ease the affected muscles, retrain posture and prove helpful with poor co-ordination. Even if you suffer from severe spasticity, passive exercise, where another person moves your limbs for you, is important each day as it helps to prevent contractures. A relaxant or pain-killer may be necessary for this to be possible but when the spasticity does ease, the limbs will return to working order much more quickly. Some find it helps to have massage or a bath before physiotherapy exercise, but avoid getting overheated.

Often it is rare that anyone gets more than one or two physiotherapy sessions per week, and then probably only for a limited period of time. Capitalize on what help is given by continuing to do the exercises at home. What you must always watch out for is not to go over your fatigue threshold. You gain greater benefit from frequent exercise in small doses than from

of finding beneficial ways of controlling its react
behind it is that once you become aware of some
can learn to control that function. It involves a ce
-awareness, and employs the techniques of yo
chnology of modern biofeedback machinery.
ntative than curative, biofeedback seems to
r MS. This probably lies with the stress factor of
cope with stress depends on recognizing s
body. Many people are never fully aware of e
ir body and struggle on in a state of partial ten
body under partial tension, they become pro
problems which may aggravate MS. Using a
ne that monitors electrical skin resistance can s
cognize body reactions to stress and warn them
lax.

scutaneous Electrical Nerve

lication of a low-level pulse electrical current
gh electrodes placed on the skin. This self-t
ular with people with MS as a means of redu
nating pain. The current apparently restricts
pain impulses while stimulating the bod
pain-relieving hormones.
widely used in hospitals and pain clinics and
arity with physiotherapists. Small, lightweight
easy to use and invaluable in the control of n
are associated with MS.

xygen (HBO)

ents some people with MS value is HBO. The
is high pressure and HBO treatment consist
en through a face mask while sitting in a n
he air pressure has been raised by pumpin
y behind the treatment is that oxygen at hi
ress inflammation around the MS diseased a
prevent its spread. Those undergoing I
not suffer from epilepsy or any heart condit
0s there was general excitement over sensati
dia of cures or considerable improvement
ment. There was a rush for places and volunt
g in the supervision of HBO chambers. Vari
true clinical value of HBO treatment have si

overtiring yourself in a work-out which it takes days to recover from.

Physiotherapy treatment is normally arranged in Britain by your GP on an out-patient appointment basis. It can be both time-consuming and exhausting to wait for transport to and from out-patient clinics and this can counteract the benefit of the actual treatment. Occasionally, however, it is possible for a physiotherapist to come to your home to treat you. Physiotherapy is also available privately.

Massage

A good massage both relaxes and stimulates. General massage improves the circulation of the blood, thus aiding the nervous and immune systems to work at peak efficiency. Massage can also focus on relieving muscle tension and spasm. An old-fashioned technique called 'cupping' applied either side of the spinal cord has proved valuable for some people with MS. Massage works well in combination with bathing first. You must expect to feel very tired after it and may need time to build up a tolerance to its undoubtedly beneficial long-term effects.

Reflexology

More than just another form of massage, reflexology can be beneficial to people with MS. It is based on the principle of the body being divided into zones, each linked to a key point on one of the feet. By massaging the appropriate area of the foot, it is possible to treat the problems in the related body zone or organ. Simple and harmless, it often produces surprising results.

Yoga

Yoga will work successfully as long as you are willing to accept some of its philosophy as well as its practice. It is not a form of treatment, but more a way of taking control of yourself and making a conscious decision to integrate body, mind and spirit into a smoothly functioning whole. If you have time for the whole person approach and are sympathetic to the concept that good health depends on harmony, balance and maintaining natural rhythms, you will discover that yoga has much to offer.

Yoga seems to provide an antidote to the tensions of MS – both the tensions that arise as a consequence of the disease itself and those that are a reaction to living with it. There's no doubt that both types of tension can build up to such an extent that people easily

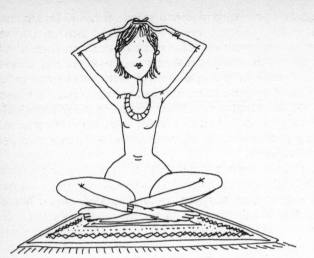

YOGA WILL WORK SUCCESSFULLY FOR YOU AS LONG
AS YOU ARE WILLING TO ACCEPT SOME OF ITS PHILOSOPHY
AS WELL AS ITS PRACTICE.

get locked into MS. Yoga counteracts this by allowing you to function fully once more, no longer fragmented but able to harness the total of what you are so that it is easier to cope. It invites you to accept life as it comes and teaches the skills to work in a systematic but relaxed way within the restrictions of the disease or problem area. It gives you a new option to choose in the place of grim determination and gritting your teeth when faced with a setback. Enthusiasts claim that yoga has much to offer that is of specific benefit to a disease like MS because it can maximize energy, give new tone to the neuromuscular system, have a positive effect on the immune system, improve the function of the glands, build up resistance to illness and keep the body supple.

Yoga teaches you how to breathe for maximum benefit so that tensions in your body are released and its energy is made fully available. The basis of energy control is knowing how to relax. During relaxation gentle diaphragmatic breathing maintains a continual flow of energy. In addition to this you need to practise specific breath control involving the diaphragm. By taking a strong breath in and then breathing out slowly, you are giving more oxygen to the body and brain and stimulating energy flow. This control of mind, body and energy is fully co-ordinated when you involve yoga movements, or asanas. Yoga movements can be done lying down, sitting on a chair or standing. Many are very simple, the more complex ones being a combination of simpler movements,

linked together with careful a
Even if you are unable to mov
visualize the movement you
breath to give you energy w
limb is also beneficial. It is of
position, but just trying to d
effect on the body. It is well v
or desire to give up, if resu
work like a key, unlocking
live better with MS.

Yoga classes are quite pop
in easily enough with a regu
remedial yoga classes desig
the disabilities of MS.

Aromatheraphy

Aromatherapists believe t
can be absorbed through th
skin, they are thought to t
seep into the bloodstream
of which may prove hea
anti-viral properties of es
infection.

Each essential oil has
an effect on both body a
Many oils seem to serv
fascinating reading to
body.

By far the best and m
massage. The reaction
endings and stimulate
skin. In any case, a goo
a good sense of well-b
warm bath. There they
are also inhaled.

Whether or not you
be no doubt that it is
Even if its beneficial
the oils, together with
gives invariably has

Biofeedback

This is a method of l

responds and
The principle
function, you
degree of self
well as the te

More preve
some value fo
The ability to
reactions in th
of stress on th
By keeping th
psychosomatic
feedback mach
them how to re
they need to r

TENS (Tra
Stimulation

TENS is the ap
the body throu
ment unit is po
and even elimi
transmission of
produce its own

TENS units ar
gaining in popul
portable, they ar
of the pains that

Hyperbaric

One of the treatm
'hyperbaric' mear
breathing in oxyg
chamber where t
oxygen. The theo
pressure can supp
of the brain and
treatment should

In the early 198
reports in the me
result of HBO trea
underwent trainin
trials to assess the

been carried out. The results of these show that there is no objective and only a little subjective benefit from HBO. This is disappointing. Nevertheless, there are still HBO chambers in operation and some people with MS do feel they benefit from a course of treatment. If HBO is used, it would be wise to check that the chamber is properly supervised and bear in mind that any positive effect is unlikely to be lasting.

Acupuncture

Acupuncture works on the principle of there being a series of points in the body, approximately 800, each linked to an organ. If an organ fails to function during an illness or spell of ill health, the point registers the dysfunction. The points are understood to be linked together in a line known as a meridian, which works as a sort of energy pathway. If the points remain in balance along their meridian, you enjoy a state of health. If there is a lack of energy, or an excess of it, the meridian becomes sensitive and registers a state of imbalance or illness.

The work of the acupuncturist is to make sure the meridians have an even flow of energy passing through them. This is achieved by using needles, the pricks of which stimulate specific nerves. The electrical impulses generated register in the brain, the spinal cord and the affected area. Needles of pure metal only are used, notably copper, silver (for a sedative effect) and gold (to stimulate). The acupuncturist knows which meridian to treat by making a pulse diagnosis, read at the wrist. It is claimed that such a diagnosis gives information about the present state of health and may even be predictive.

Acupuncture should not be viewed as a panacea for all ills, but as a treatment that has proved useful over a wide therapeutic range and one that often combines well with other therapies. It may help to alleviate some symptoms of MS such as pain, spasms, pins and needles, tingling sensations, and coldness in limbs. Too often, however, the relief experienced is only temporary and the symptoms treated are likely to reappear.

Hydrotherapy

Water is a natural and thorough cleansing agent, internally as well as externally. Although not much in fashion today, it is still much valued by natural therapists. In continental Europe it is still common for people with MS to be treated with hydrotherapy at clinics in spa towns.

There is no one correct way to bathe because everybody has such

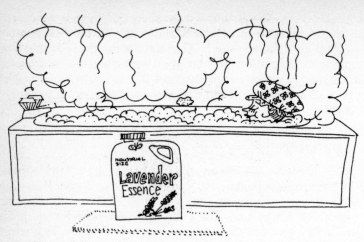

THERE IS GREAT ADVANTAGE IN RELAXING AND UNWINDING
IN A BATH, PERHAPS WITH ESSENCES OF PINE AND LAVENDER,
SO GOOD FOR THE NERVOUS SYSTEM.

different skin. Showering may be preferable to bathing. The
circulation will be stimulated by showering with cold and warm
water alternately. However, there is great advantage to relaxing
and unwinding in a bath, perhaps with essences of pine or
lavender, so good for the nervous system. Not only are tense
muscles eased but the psychological effect is very beneficial.

It may be necessary for bathing to be supervised initially, as it is
common with MS to feel weak afterwards, until a healthy resistance
to it has been built up. When that happens, hydrotherapy can give
energy as well as a sense of well-being.

Hippotherapy

Hippotherapy is horse-riding for treatment as well as pleasure. It is
particularly encouraged as a treatment for MS in Switzerland and
Scandinavia because it provides gentle exercise for the muscles,
improves co-ordination and concentration, and is a socially
approved pastime.

Nutrition and diets

What you eat makes a difference to how healthy you are. Bodies fed
only junk food overwork. They struggle to cope with the longer and
more complex process of digesting 'junk' and scratch around more
to extract the wholesome nutrition they require to function well.

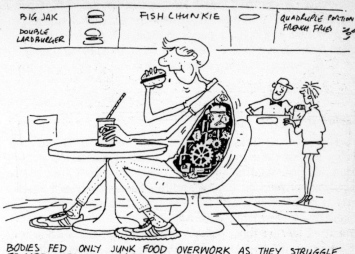

BIG JAK
DOUBLE LARDBURGER
FISH CHUNKIE
QUADRUPLE PORTION FRENCH FRIES

BODIES FED ONLY JUNK FOOD OVERWORK AS THEY STRUGGLE TO COPE WITH THE LONGER AND MORE COMPLEX PROCESS OF DIGESTING 'JUNK'

The healthiest diets include fresh, natural and unprocessed foods – salads, fruits and vegetables, whole grains, nuts and pulses, white fish, chicken, limited amounts of lean red meat, small quantities of dairy products, few eggs and plenty of water. These foods are absorbed easily and broken down efficiently to give you the energy you need. Information like this has had a positive impact on diet in general and even many convenience foods are prepared healthily.

The best diet for MS must not only be normally healthy but, in addition, compensate for any deficiencies in the nervous and immune systems of the body. Since research shows that levels of saturated fats are higher and levels of polyunsaturated fats lower than average in people with MS, the importance of a low-fat diet has been stressed. This is also in line with what is best for the immune system, whose lymphatic system is responsible for fighting invasion. A high-fat diet thickens and clogs up the lymph, so fatty foods are best avoided. Adequate protein is important, as are vitamins and minerals, which occur naturally in fresh fruits, salads, vegetables, nuts, grains and seeds. For example, vitamin C, found in good supply in oranges, kiwis and green peppers, helps attack viral and bacterial infection. The B vitamins – B_5, B_6, B_{12} and folic acid – are similarly important. Vitamins A and E help protect cells from damage. Minerals such as calcium, magnesium, selenium and zinc are needed. Zinc, in particular, has a significant effect on the body's immune responses.

Although no one diet has been proved to cure MS, there are strong indications that a low-fat diet with additional sunflower oil and vitamins E and A has a very beneficial effect long term. There is a scientific basis for this. Other diets sometimes recommended are more to do with personal preference, individual taste and circumstantial evidence.

Low-fat diets

A diet low in saturated fats is strongly advised. Dietary fat is *probably* the single most important nutrient associated with MS. Epidemiological studies since the 1950s have indicated a strong association between dietary fat and MS. Saturated fat rich foods are clearly correlated with MS while polyunsaturated fatty rich foods are negatively associated with MS.

Saturated fats are those solid at room temperature such as butter, lard and coconut and avocado oils. These are unnecessary in the diet as the body has no problem in producing saturated fats by converting other food sources. This is untrue of unsaturated fats, which the body alone cannot produce enough of. Therefore it is wise to supplement your diet with unsaturated fats such as sunflower, safflower or evening primrose oils. Sunflower oil supplements have been shown in scientific tests to produce a clear reduction in both the relapse rates of MS and the severity of the disease. Unsaturated fats are soft or liquid at room temperature and contain three essential fatty acids which may be significant in MS. These are linoleic acid its converted form gammalinolenic acid and arachidonic acid. They are vital to the healthy functioning of the body. People with MS are known to have low levels of linoleic and arachidonic acid in their blood cells and body fluids, a deficiency that appears to respond to correction by diet. Many foods provide rich sources of these acids – nuts (especially walnuts and brazils), green-leafed vegetables and salads (the darker the green the better), green peppers, bean sprouts, carrots, wheatgerm, fruits (including tomatoes), soyabeans, poultry and white fish (such as cod, mackerel, salmon and sardines). Essential fatty acids are needed for brain growth and the development of the central nervous system, including the repair of myelin. Any deficiency in them has a negative effect on the function and maintenance of the body. As vitamins C and E are anti-oxidant agents preventing the destruction of unsaturated fatty acids, you should ensure you have sufficient of these too.

Allergy reactions

It is possible for MS-type symptoms to be experienced because of an allergy problem. Cutting out what you are allergic to is the basis of several much publicized diets. The Swank diet cuts out sugar and the Evers diet recommends huge quantities of fresh fruit and vegetables, grains and a very low-fat intake. The MacDougall and Rita Greer diets are basically gluten-free, low in sugar, low in saturated fat and abundant in fruits, vegetables and pulses. They were devised for Roger MacDougall and Roger Greer, who maintained they had recovered from their MS symptoms as a direct result.

There is ample evidence that some people are especially sensitive to certain foods. Common foods that many people with MS appear allergic to are dairy products, yeast in foods, mushrooms, fermented products (such as vinegar), sugar, potatoes and tea. If you think you may be allergic to any foods or chemicals, you should get tested for this. This can be done by going on a total or cleansing fast first and then testing out various foods. Alternatively there are doctors trained in nutrition and clinical ecologists who offer food allergy testing for a fee.

Exercise and diet

Any diet works best when it is co-ordinated with exercise and getting sufficient relaxation and deep sleep. Getting enough exercise when you have MS may be difficult, but even ten minutes a day is beneficial. The lymph, the carrier of immune cells round the body, keeps on the move because of muscular contraction provided by movement. Even if you cannot jog or do aerobics, gentler types of exercise and massage can be effective too. Exercise will also aid the digestion, enabling you to benefit fully from the food you eat.

Suggestions for healthy eating

- Keep meals simple and low fat:
  – plan main meals on a basis of brown rice, wholemeal pasta or jacket potatoes.
  – add a minimal amount of protein in the form of fish, poultry, small portions of lean red meat, an egg or two occasionally, low-fat cheese or pulses (lentils, beans or soya products, which are not gaseous if you add a little wine to the cooking).
  – make sure you have enough raw salads and lightly-cooked vegetables. Include sprouting seeds which are a rich source of vitamins and minerals.

- Avoid rich, fatty, sugary, over-refined and over-processed foods.
- Learn to enjoy natural foods.
- Increase your fluid intake, especially of pure water (up to 2 litres a day).
- Whenever possible use:
  skimmed or semi-skimmed milk
  low-fat natural yoghurt
  a margarine high in polyunsaturates such as a sunflower one
  low-fat cheese, eg cottage, low-fat Cheddar, Edam, Gouda
  fresh fish, skinned poultry and lean meats – grilled, steamed, poached
  jacket, boiled, steamed or mashed potatoes
  2–3 eggs per week
  wholemeal flour products and brown rice
  fresh foods, especially plenty of salads and fresh fruit – all the brightly coloured vegetables are particularly healthy.
- Eat as much raw food as possible and only lightly cook green vegetables.

Oils: Sunflower, safflower and evening primrose

Many studies have shown that linoleic and arachidonic acids, two essential fatty acids, are low in the blood cells and body fluids of people with MS. Essential fatty acids may also be required as the building blocks for the repair of myelin. It is also possible that a metabolic abnormality in the unsaturated fatty acid metabolism exists. This fortunately appears to be responsive to diet. Sunflower supplements to the diets of people with MS have consistently shown a reduction in the relapse rate and severity of the disease. In people mildly affected by MS there was an apparent decrease in the long-term progression of the disease. It would seem that the addition of at least 20 grams of sunflower oil per day is of positive value.

For similar reasons many people with MS take oil of evening primrose capsules as a valuable dietary supplement and credit this oil with producing an overall improvement, even if there is limited scientific evidence to back it. The North American Indians first used this small plant with bright yellow flowers for medicinal purposes. They found it had great powers of healing, particularly against skin conditions and infections. Today the evening primrose is valued for its high content of gamma-linolenic acid or GLA, essential for health and easily converted into prostaglandin I. All prostaglandins keep an up-to-the-second check on the working of every cell in the body. Prostaglandin I, the end result of both evening primrose oil, and the even richer safflower oil has special responsibility for the blood. With MS the fact that prostaglandins ensure enough T-lymphocytes to fight infection may be significant. There is evidence from other auto-immune diseases that the use of a low-fat diet and essential fatty acid supplements such as sunflower safflower and evening primrose oils are beneficial.

Smoking, alcohol and MS

Smoking

As so many doctors shrug their shoulders when asked if it is all right to smoke if you have MS, they obviously operate on the principle that anything that gives pleasure and temporary relief is worthwhile, even if it actually does harm. However, there is ample evidence that smoking is harmful in general and that it has particularly negative effects on MS.

When you smoke, you inhale carbon monoxide, which forms a fixed and irreversible combination with the haemoglobin in your blood. This has two effects. Firstly the blood thickens and circulation is reduced. The central nervous system requires healthy blood circulation. The other effect is that the blood can no longer take up oxygen so easily and you experience breathlessness as a result. If MS has reduced your mobility, your breathing capacity has already been lowered. Add the effects of smoking to this and you are more likely to suffer from bronchitis and pneumonia.

Cigarettes and cigars produce a number of poisonous by-products. One of these is nicotine, which has a powerful effect interrupting the transmission of messages along the nerve pathways. Cyanide is another poison, not produced in dangerous quantities, but enough to cause some negative effect.

Smoking also has a pronounced effect on the peripheral nerves, putting them under pressure. For example, if you already have trouble with opening the bladder, the problem will be aggravated because smoking strengthens the bladder's sphincter, the muscle responsible for keeping the bladder shut.

Alcohol

Alcohol has a noticeable effect on the central nervous system too. A poison to the nerves affecting their normal function, it is a strong suppresser of the immune system. Excessive drinking progressively weakens the immune system. People with MS may find that they have to reduce the number of drinks they have because they become 'legless' sooner than they used to.

Counselling

Counselling gives you an opportunity to explore in a safe, understanding, professional relationship what it means for you to live with MS. It is difficult to cope with the way MS interferes in your life. If you have the disease, you may find its existence and symptoms so intrusive and frightening that the need to express what it is like is the only bit of relief you can get. Yet talking about it as much as you need to will bore and frustrate most people, even those nearest and dearest. If you don't have MS yourself but are close to someone who has, you too deserve space to express your own reactions and needs. In both instances, talking things through in confidence with a trained counsellor will allow you to face the experience of MS, and discover the resources still within you and the support available from others.

As each person's needs are different, the counsellor uses his or her skills to focus on you and create the right environment for you to discover for yourself in your own way and time what contributes to or blocks your coping well with MS. It is to do with unlocking your own inner strengths and resources, which seem to go under wraps when anything like a chronic illness comes on the scene. You need understanding support before you can accept how normal it is with MS to experience strong emotional reactions, to doubt your own self-worth and to wonder what useful contribution you can make to the world. Inevitably, you will have to reappraise your relationships at home, at work and socially, and face the fact of a less certain future. Through counselling you can choose to face and learn to like yourself. This is a rewarding enough experience in itself. Even more relevant and exciting is the added bonus of an improvement in health. It has been said of MS that few diseases are so positively affected by good emotional health. The wholeness that comes from learning to accept yourself is the result expected of successful counselling. While it is true that the love, acceptance and understanding of someone close to you produces the most wonderfully enriching and empowering relationship, few can combine such intimacy with the impartiality needed for personal growth in the other.

Some people suppose that only a counsellor who has first-hand experience of MS can counsel someone with the disease. This is not so. The work of the counsellor is not to swap personal experiences of MS, which is the strength of a self-help group, but to allow you to discover the facts of MS and how to maximize your life with it. It is important that you and your counsellor are well informed about MS, but your personal reactions to it are the stuff of counselling. Obviously it is essential for every counsellor to appreciate, for example, the strength and pervasiveness of MS fatigue or the way in which demyelination can affect general mood. However, it is likely that emotional blocks aggravate these symptoms and resolving the blocks releases energy for healing and coping better with life.

Your GP will be able to refer you to a counsellor or clinical psychologist or you can make your own arrangements. A counselling session usually lasts for one hour once a week over an agreed period of time. There are many different kinds of counselling, all of them with their merits, but what matters most is that you feel at ease with the counsellor, who should have experience and be in supervision. Trust your own gut reactions and allow your reactions to the first interview to determine whether to go ahead with this counsellor on a regular basis or have an interview with a different one. The booklet 'Is It For Me?', published by the British Association of Counselling is very informative.

Hypnotherapy

Hypnosis does not treat symptoms so much as look at the causes of ill-health. A fully-trained hypnotherapist looks at the whole person and helps you through hypnosis to speak freely about your feelings and emotions. When hypnosis works well you will find symptoms may disappear or be reducing as you relax and become aware of your inner self. It is frequently the quickest and most effective method of discovering what pressures you have been under and getting free of them, which would certainly be beneficial if you have MS. On the other hand, it may never work or be a technique you regard with suspicion.

Self-help groups

Self-help groups are a way of dealing with problems of all kinds by talking them over with others who have gone through a similar experience. Self-help is a way of reaching outside of yourself, acknowledging your right to get support and believing that others have something to give you. It helps you live through today and have the courage to want to live tomorrow too.

Self-help is not a panacea for all ills, but just one of many ways of coping with MS. Instead of being 'done to', being on the receiving end of treatment, advice and care, you become actively involved in a unique process of sharing. In talking about your experience of MS with others who also have it, you give each other mutual support.

Self-help groups are generally small groups and informal. The focus of the help is on the individual and his or her needs. Who you are and your personal experience of life and MS are what count. It is not always what you say or do not say that makes an impression. The fact that you want to be there to give yourself and others a chance to share is all important.

Financial help

You may be entitled to some form of financial assistance, because of difficulties caused by MS. Many of the organizations listed in the Useful Addresses section can give further information about this.
Benefits a person with MS may be entitled to receive are:

Attendance Allowance
Disability Living Allowance (with Care and Mobility components)
Disability Working Allowance
Family Credit
Housing Benefit and Council Tax Benefit
Incapacity Benefit
Income Support
Invalid Care Allowance
Job Seekers Allowance
Severe Disablement Allowance
Sickness Benefit
Social Fund
Statutory Sick Pay

People with a disability and their carers have a right to have their needs assessed for the social services available under Section 2 of the Chronically Sick and Disabled Persons Act of 1970. These specifically include:

aids and adaptations
holidays
meals at home or at a local centre
outings, games and excursions – and transport to and from such activities
practical help in the home
respite care
telephones and any special equipment needed to use the phone
television, radio or library facilities

Carers are now being given long-overdue recognition for their tireless support and the Carers (Recognition and Services) Act 1995 is designed to be of assistance to them.

Trends in MS research

Back to the puzzle

The complexity of MS has already been pictured in this book as a giant jigsaw puzzle. What some of those pieces are and how they fit together, or at least appear to belong in roughly the same area, and how current research fits in will be explored here.

The sort of questions that people with MS want answers to are simple. However, as the human body is so complex, and the study of its biology and the way it works still only understood in part, even the names of the various branches of science involved in MS research sound baffling, let alone their fields of study. The pieces of the jigsaw thought to be at the centre of the puzzle are the fields of basic and clinical immunology and the biology of glia, with neurophysiology, virology and genetics adjacent, and psychosocial aspects, rehabilitation and ways of improving diagnosis completing the structure. Until the cause of MS becomes clear, everyone with an interest in the disease, personal as well as professional, seems under a compulsion to return to the jigsaw again and again, just to see if they can fit in a piece of the puzzle that no one else has noticed, the piece that will make all the difference. Everyone wants a cure for MS. If you live with it, more practical answers become urgent when you find your life disrupted by its symptoms.

A historical framework

It seems reasonable to start by clarifying the historical development of MS research as a framework. MS has been known as a disease since the mid nineteenth century and it was described as such by Charcot in 1868, though it was previously identified by the Scot, Carswell. Although classified then, MS has remained so mysterious that efforts to cure, treat or manage it have had to cover a wide range of possibilities.

It was first thought to have resulted from overexertion and total rest was prescribed. Then suspicion fell on some sort of infection or inflammation that would presumably respond to vaccines, antibiotics or even blood transfusions. From the start there was interest in complementary therapies to make good any damage, and the areas of nutrition and diets, vitamin supplements and desensitization were explored. So too were certain psychiatric techniques such as hypnosis.

With the widespread use of objective diagnostic tests, MS is no longer confused with hysteria, a diagnosis some women received in the recent past. In the 1920s MS could only be proved by post-mortem tissue examination. Rehabilitation was worked at and treatments, including various types of massage and electrical stimulation of the spinal cord, were tried to ease the symptoms. Any avenue of research and treatment was followed, however remote its connection or significance to MS.

The global perspective

As in the past, so today every area of scientific and medical knowledge is eagerly scanned, no longer simply for pointers to a cause and cure for MS, but more for further pieces of the puzzle.

If the outer edge of the jigsaw puzzle is the historical perspective, the pieces that fit next to the edge form the global overview that is obtained from epidemiological studies. Epidemiological research is the study of populations for certain kinds of data: who they are in terms of race and origin; where they live in terms of latitude, environment and climate; and how they live in terms of livelihood, hygiene, nutrition and diet. Such studies can focus on a particular group of people over a limited time period, or an extended (or longitudinal) survey covering several generations. It is epidemiological investigation that unearths clues and suggests directions to be followed up by researchers in other disciplines. The everyday sort of questions that we ask about MS fall within the sphere of epidemiologists. Who gets MS? Is there an equal chance of getting MS irrespective of where you live? Does it make any difference if you are born and grow up in one region and then move to another in adulthood? When do people get MS? What links are there between MS and the environment?

Epidemiology has already shown that the patterns of MS vary from one racial group to another and thus paves the way for analytical research to be done by geneticists. Also uncovered by epidemiologists has been evidence suggesting the involvement of a virus or other agent in MS, comparisons between the high prevalence of MS in the cool temperate zones, most especially in the north and among those of Nordic stock, and its apparent absence near the equator and poles, and documentary evidence from areas with a high MS population and the one 'epidemic' of MS on the Faroe Islands after the Second World War.

The fact that MS is often found in regional clusters does not suggest that an environmental cause is very likely but rather that genetic isolates must exist. The cause is more likely to do with who lives where than with where they live. For example, there seems to be an over-representation of susceptibility genes in the Orkneys and Shetlands and an absence of them in the Hutterite communities of North America. Migration studies show that the risk of developing MS in a single ethnic group varies according to the place of residence during a critical period of childhood. Data on black Africans moving to the USA suggests that the risk of MS correlates with the introduction of Caucasian genes into the black community. An increased risk of MS in white populations is linked with genes that code for products involved in the immune response to extrinsic antigens.

Also documented by epidemiologists is the personal experience of people with MS – how they cope, the effects of MS on their lifestyle and the typical progression of the disease. This type of information enables doctors and health care specialists to understand better how to manage MS and best support those with it.

The multi-factorial nature of MS

What do they think MS is?

There is general agreement that MS appears to be an auto-immune disease, triggered by environmental factors in individuals who have a genetic susceptibility. An auto-immune disease is one in which the body's immune system mistakenly attacks its own healthy cells or tissue instead of going for a foreign invader such as a virus or bacterium. In MS the attack concentrates on myelin. Auto-immunity may be the cause of the destruction of the myelin but the fact that triggers and genetic susceptibility are involved means that MS has to be considered a *multi-factorial disease* – that is, a disease that can be caused by a combination of many different factors. Each factor has to be investigated separately for specific information to do with MS. An example of this would be the composition, function and the processes of myelin breakdown and rebuilding (demyelination and remyelination). Discovering more about what myelin is leads to further questions as to why myelin gets attacked, what triggers the attack, whether it can be stopped and the damage repaired. Thus the knock-on effect of investigating myelin leads to the involvement of other specialized sciences that overlap or interconnect.

Why don't they know the cause of MS?

The quick answer is that MS is highly complex. In order to

understand disease mechanisms, fact is tested against theory, a creative, intricate and painstaking process. MS research, the main focus of which is bio-medical, has to involve a host of projects so detailed and specialized that communication between researchers, far from happening automatically, has to be co-ordinated for it to happen at all. Fortunately communication barriers between researchers are reduced at world symposia on current research into MS.

Perhaps the key event is organized by the International Federation of MS Societies (IFMSS), which has a membership of 34 national societies and whose research symposia attract researchers world-wide. A primary aim of the IFMSS is to stimulate scientific and medical research relating to MS as well as serving as a central clearing-house for educational information on the disease. Only by sharing the latest research can the cause and thus the cure of the disease be found.

Who does the research and who pays?

MS societies around the world fund a host of research projects specific to MS in a search for its cause, viable treatments, better diagnosis and cure. If you look at what MS research is currently being carried out around the world, around three-quarters is funded from within the United States, almost a tenth from the United Kingdom and the remainder from the rest of the world. Half of the money spent on MS research in Europe is funded from the United Kingdom. In the first half of the 1990s the number of MS research projects in the United Kingdom doubled, approximately two thirds funded by the MS Society and one third by science foundations and others.

To take the specific example of the United Kingdom: the MS Society works through its MS Medical Research Advisory Committee, made up of experts in their fields. Their brief is to fund only the top priority projects, which must be clearly relevant to MS. The committee is also responsible for monitoring the progress of these projects and for ensuring that the results are made known. The thirst for the latest information on research is insatiable.

The value of MRI scanning

MRI (magnetic resonance imaging) scanning is by far the most important advance in the investigation of MS. MRI scanners are safe to use on a regular basis and sensitive enough to pick out areas of lesions in the brain and spinal cord. They are like a window, allowing researchers to view what is happening in the central nervous system. Thus they are helpful (but not always necessary) for diagnostic purposes, and invaluable for the prediction of MS and monitoring the results of clinical trials. It is now possible to determine whether people with MS who get fewer symptoms while undergoing clinical trials are improving because they are in remission or because of the treatment.

When MRI scanning was first used, it was expected that the close observation of inflammation and demyelination would reveal a definite correlation between what was seen on the scans and the actual disability suffered by the person with MS. This has not proved to be the case. The number and size of lesions does not always correlate with the visible symptoms. However, by using new technology such as MR spectroscopy, MRI scanners can detect not only very early changes in myelin and identify lesions at different stages of development but also focus in on damage that extends beyond the myelin. There is a strong likelihood that the severity of the disability that accompanies the primary progressive form of MS is a result of damage to the actual nerve fibres/axons, in addition to the regular damage to the myelin sheath.

What types of MS research are being carried out?

Bio-medical research. Firstly there is basic scientific research in order to understand what MS is, what causes it and ultimately how to cure it. The biology of glial cells, which form myelin, is the prime example of this. There are two types of cell resident in the brain: *nerve* and *glial*. The glial cells are *astrocytes*, responsible for the structure; *oligodendrocytes*, which make the myelin; and *microglia*, whose task is to remove any debris. As more is understood about myelin, it seems increasingly likely that damaged myelin may be repaired or regenerated (remyelination). This may be made feasible by cultivating oligodendrocytes for transplantation and programming them via genetic engineering to go to the scattered areas of damage in MS. The implications of such promising research are how to overcome the difficulty in obtaining sufficient oligodendrocytes (most plentiful in foetal or other suitable biopsy tissue), but which may also be grown in the laboratory. Another example of basic scientific research is the fundamental processes of nerve growth and development, vital to research in any disease of the central nervous system.

The major area of current MS research is in the area of immunology. The nature of auto-immunity is fundamental to all research into central nervous system diseases. Advances in such research in the last decade indicate that it is now possible to do something about neuro-genetic diseases. In MS it is vital to understand the attacking cells better and how they move from the blood to the brain. How do such destructive cells fool the blood-brain barrier into letting them through? If they could be stopped from getting into the central nervous system in the first place, MS would be prevented in people at risk of developing the disease. Alternatively, if they do slip through, another preventative measure would be to stop them from attacking myelin. The idea of exterminating the attacking cells before they cause demyelination may sound like something in a child's video game but it is one option.

The other options – finding ways to suppress or alter the immune system – could also lead to the development of new treatments for MS.

Data gathered from epidemiological studies suggests that some environmental factor may be important in triggering MS. This is thought likely to be a virus, although no single virus has been linked with MS. If there were a virus, then a vaccine could be developed.

Advances in genetics are showing that many diseases are caused by a single defective gene. This is not considered to be likely for MS but there is sufficient evidence to suggest that a complex combination of certain normal genes makes a person prone to developing MS. A positive outcome would be if those, especially children, susceptible to developing MS later in life could be identified genetically. Then some new therapeutic strategies could be developed.

Psychosocial and rehabilitation research.   Research into how best to live with MS and what type of support people with MS and their families need is vital too. This is achieved in two ways: through research projects that will survey general and specific needs, and also through individual practical support.

Areas of research in more detail
The role of myelin

As already explained in Chapter 1, damage to myelin, the protective sheath around axons in the central nervous system, has a negative effect on the transmission of nerve impulses, slowing it down so much that MS symptoms appear as a consequence. The build-up of scar tissue in the place of myelin is another reason for MS symptoms, because the nerve impulses cannot function as normal. So one major research goal is to find agents that can stimulate the repair of myelin.

Two types of glial cells in the brain cells support the nerve cells and produce myelin. The oligodendrocytes produce nerve-insulating myelin and if their function is understood, it should be possible to find ways of repairing MS damage. The astrocytes play a destructive role by rapidly generating scar tissue along damaged nerve fibres and maybe even block myelin repair. It would help to know what triggers induce scar tissue formation and then it would be possible to find ways of preventing scarring and allowing myelin regeneration. A particular focus of research is on the role of *cytokines*, chemical messengers involved in the destruction of myelin. If ways of stimulating the regrowth of myelin can be found, neurological function could be restored in people with MS.

The natural process of remyelination involves both progenitor cells and oligodendrocytes, which migrate to wherever in the brain needs to be remyelinated. In some cases this can occur so quickly and successfully that lesions may disappear. This is not always so, however, as sometimes the development of some lesions outstrips the attempt to remyelinate. Such lesions become permanent and contain non-myelinating cells in a process called gliosis.

Oligodendrocyte progenitor cells are now being grown with the prospect of being transplanted into the brain for the purpose of remyelination. It is hoped that such cells will be accepted by the human brain and the progression of MS gradually halted and in the long term reversed.

Demyelination or inflammation?

The basic cause of MS is to do with demyelination and inflammation, but which comes first has not always been clear. Either primary inflammation leads to demyelination or it results alongside myelin products being broken down in some other way. Evidence now points to inflammation as the primary factor because under experimental conditions, auto-immune demyelination is dependent on the inflammation mechanism. This appears to be confirmed by observations on patients with the use of the MRI scanner, whose enhanced pictures can pick out details that include the presence of inflammation.

Immunology

What is the normal function of the immune system

The immune system is a highly complex system of defence against infection. It does this by means of antibodies or immune T-cells to deal with what it sees as an invader to be wiped out. The warning that an invader has breached defences is given by antigens.

Antigens are complex molecules on the surface of cells, which the immune system either recognizes as 'self' and ignores or fails to recognize and attacks the cell as alien. A vital function of the healthy immune system is to recognize itself and not destroy its own tissue by mistake. Virtually all aspects of the regulation of the immune system are investigated in MS research.

Multiple sclerosis and auto-immunity

What is thought to happen in MS is that there is a specific malfunctioning of the immune system – an abnormal auto-immune response. One way in which the immune system can malfunction is to misidentify its own tissue. In MS the immune system malfunctions by directing the T-cells to destroy the healthy protein component of the myelin sheath. It is as if a misdirected attack has been launched on myelin in the brain and spinal cord, just as though the myelin were a foreign invader such as a virus or bacterium to be wiped out. This sort of self-destruct mechanism resulting from an over-active immune system is known as *auto-immunity*. However, there is still a lack of information in general about the origins of auto-immune disease.

The all-important question is 'Why?' Discovering what originally triggers the immune system to attack nerve tissue is the key to stopping MS. Should a specific antigen that triggers MS be identified, it could be used to develop a vaccine or immune-system modifier to halt the disease. It may be possible in future that people with MS will be given 'allergy shots' to desensitize the antigen. Copolymer-1 has already been used this way (see p. 106), but has produced only modest benefit in the relapsing-remitting type of MS and no positive effect in the progressive type. Another approach would be to isolate some mechanism that would neutralize the rogue T-cells hostile to myelin, reprogrammed to attack certain of its protein components. Would it be possible to disarm/inactivate the T-cells and leave the rest of the immune system intact? A different option would be to train the immune system via oral desensitization to desensitize the immune system by giving myelin antigens by mouth, so that it would 'ignore' the nerve-insulating myelin it would otherwise attack.

Getting across the blood-brain barrier

A critical step in MS is the movement of the immune cells from the bloodstream into the brain and spinal fluid. This happens when destructive immune cells are drawn to the blood-brain barrier, which normally protects the brain and spinal cord from such cells. If the factors that allow the immune cells to penetrate the blood-brain barrier can be stopped, then it is likely that inflammation and myelin destruction will be prevented.

The involvement of cytokines

Cytokines are chemicals that have an intricate regulatory/modulating interaction with immune cells. It seems that they can either assist in the destruction of myelin by helping to maintain the inflammation that precedes demyelination or do quite the opposite and protect myelin against attack by T-cells. Cytokines are certainly in evidence in the spinal fluid and lesions during an attack. Their function has been described as being responsible for taking messages. If those messages could be manipulated, then it is probable that aggressive attack could be turned off and the auto-immune response stopped. Parallel research into the receptors that encourage the cell to take notice of the cytokines involves examining the gene(s) that control the receptors. The end result desired is to understand the fundamental processes that lead to MS and to find ways of shutting down inflammation.

How does EAE help in MS research?

Experimental allergic encephalomyelitis, or EAE, is an MS-type disease induced in laboratory animals as a disease model. This approach permits immunologists to manipulate the immune system in ways that would be impossible in humans and as a result to understand more about its importance in maintaining health and its involvement in myelin-destroying disease. This type of research has provided significant information about the relationship between specific immune mechanisms and demyelination and will hopefully lead to the more precise use of immunosuppressive agents at the early stages of the disease.

Stress and the immune system

Other research has investigated the effect of stress on immune system disorders. In response to stress, the sympathetic nervous system and adrenal glands produce hormones that alert and activate the body to respond. Subsequently corticol (a corticosteroid) is produced to release glucose to sustain energy for fight or flight. It has, for example, been found that people with MS have abnormally high levels of receptors produced in response to stress.

These receptors normally suppress unwelcome immune responses. People with MS have been found to have three or four times the average number of receptors. As yet the reason for this is unclear, but it points to some malfunction between the immune and nervous systems. This link has been confirmed by animal studies and suggests a possible way in which MS attacks are caused. It may be that the abnormality in the receptors is genetically determined.

Until researchers can explain in detail how the complex regulatory processes of the immune system are damaged in MS, there will be no sure way of treating the damage. The guiding principle of immunotherapy must be to maintain a balance between controlling the disease and not stopping the immune system from fighting infection normally.

Virology

There is sufficient epidemiological evidence to suspect that the MS process may be initiated by a virus, probably one or more of the common viral infections of childhood, such as measles or mumps. No one virus has been found to be the obvious culprit. In adulthood this viral component to MS is thought to trigger the auto-immune response that destroys myelin, but only in people with a genetic susceptibility to MS. In addition increased amounts of viral particles, antibodies to various viruses, especially measles and herpes simplex type 1, and other signs of viral infection have been found in the cerebrospinal fluid (CSF) of many people with MS. It is important to stress that the possible virus component to MS is not at all contagious in the normal way; its effect is restricted within the body, where it may affect the brain and/or the body's immune cells.

The way most common viruses work is to infect and produce inflammation and tissue damage, before they are attacked and destroyed by the body's natural defence mechanisms. This happens in diseases other than MS. It is still unclear whether the presence of viruses helps to cause MS or is coincidental. A virus might act directly on the central nervous system and damage myelin or it might act more indirectly. Examples of indirect action might include a virus triggering off an auto-immune response, or injury to the central nervous system by a viral agent, or even the possibility that a virus confuses the central nervous system so much that the CNS allows another virus in. On the other hand, the immune system may mistakenly attack the brain because some component of the nerve-insulating myelin sheath closely resembles the virus or because the virus itself persists in dormant state in the brain.

Alternatively, myelin attack could represent an abnormal continuation of what was initially a normal immune response to an invading virus. The attack of the immune system on the wrong harmless target may be because it 'recognizes' some component of myelin that resembles a part of a virus. Clearly research must continue in order to find out how viruses could be involved. Then it may be possible to vaccinate against the virus and so prevent any chain reaction.

Genetics

Why me? Why my son or daughter, my brother or sister, my mother or father? Why do some people get MS and others not? What are my chances of getting MS if I am related to someone with it? Are the genetic factors of MS passed on from generation to generation?

To answer the last question first, the news is good: children of MS parents have a 99 per cent likelihood of staying free of MS. MS is not believed to be hereditary. The genetic background of MS appears to set the stage for MS rather than cause it to happen: only some people predisposed to MS will develop it. In addition, an environmental factor, still unspecified, has to be added to the genetic predisposition.

However, there is a higher than average familial link, evident from studies of the blood and tissue of relatives. Genetic research has shown that MS is six to eight times more frequent in brothers and sisters and two to four times more common in parents of people with the condition. There is also a substantially higher risk of an identical twin getting MS than for a fraternal twin or non-twin brother or sister. If you have a brother, sister or fraternal twin with MS, the likelihood of your also developing MS is just over 2 per cent but this figure rises to 26 per cent with an identical twin. Another fact is that daughters, not sons, of MS mothers are slightly more likely to develop MS. The same is not true for either sons or daughters of MS fathers. The risk of developing MS in the population as a whole is around 0.1 per cent. Information such as this is arrived at via studies of large numbers of relatives of those with MS and span several generations. It provides facts which at least put you in the picture and enable you to make intelligent choices, although at the same time they may be alarming on a personal level.

Other genetics research is arrived at via laboratory studies of genes and how they function. Specific links between childhood illnesses and genetic factors, for example, can sometimes provide a parallel for what may be happening in MS. Experimental work on animals – such as the so-called 'transgenic mouse', born with a deficient myelin sheath – should lead to a better grasp of what genetic factors control myelination and demyelination. Animal models also seem to point to several genetic factors having some control over the occurrence of MS, its pattern and severity.

The fact that certain races and ethnic groups rarely, if ever, develop MS, is now thought to be due more to their genetic inheritance than some quirk of geographical location. It was formerly assumed that living near the poles or the equator protected you against MS, and that was why Eskimos and African Bantu peoples were free of the disease. Only after gypsies had similarly been found to be free of MS, and genetic studies into these three groups undertaken, did the picture become clearer. These groups do seem to have a different 'gene pool' from the Caucasians (white races) of northern European extraction. In a similar way the Chinese and Japanese have a low incidence of MS. Even among Caucasians, there are a few isolated groups free of MS, a notable example being the Hutterite religious sect already mentioned.

Thus one line of genetic research is to find a so-called 'genetic' marker to identify people who are most at risk of developing MS. The fact that people with MS carry HLA groups A3, B7, DR2 and DQw1 more often than the general population suggests there could be a really specific genetic marker for MS.

Molecular biology is moving towards isolating specific genes that correlate with the different characteristics of MS. Molecular geneticists are seeking the specific chromosomes, genes and gene structures relating to the potential for developing MS. If a gene susceptibility to MS is found, then it will be possible to develop treatment to correct the basic defect that permits the condition to occur. An example of this is monoclonal antibody therapy, which would depend on identification of a particular T-cell or antigen, and which may offer a specific treatment for MS in the future.

Related areas of research

Conduction

MS symptoms such as vision problems, memory impairment, paralysis and numbness are the result of disruptions in the transmission of electrical signals along nerve fibres in the brain and spinal cord. In remission, when remyelination takes place, conduction is restored but is still slowed down and so another focus of research is on what other factors contribute to the conduction block.

It is important to find out more about how inflammation interferes with the conduction of nerve messages. If researchers are to find ways to correct nerve signal malfunctions in MS, it is also vital to understand how healthy nerves work.

Here again, evoked potential testing and the enhanced MRI pictures are useful. They make it more possible to explore how inflammation interferes with conduction.

Another line of investigation is the way in which the disease process of MS interferes with the transmission of the electrical code. It is possible for conduction to be restored in blocked nerve fibres in acute lesions using corticosteroids, the effect of these drugs being to reverse the increased permeability of the blood-brain barrier, at least temporarily. Chronic lesions, however, are not so easily affected because of the greater damage in varying degrees to different nerve fibres. Each fibre responds differently to the steroids with the potential of distorting rather than restoring harmony to the transmission of messages along nerve pathways. Thus, as corticosteroid treatment is non-specific in nature, it is of limited benefit. In addition, it can produce some unpleasant side-effects, such as adrenal suppression, water retention, diabetes, loss of bone mineral, muscle bulk, thinning of the skin, a 'moon' face, mental disturbances, ulcers, acne and susceptibility to infection.

The vascular system

It is possible that a poor supply of blood to the tissues might contribute to the formation of lesions. It has been found that small blood vessels tend to get blocked around some MS lesions. Also some abnormalities in blood-clotting have been noticed in some persons with MS. Research continues to discover how sensitive to MS an inadequate blood supply is and, if so, to suggest what should be done to improve it.

Precipitating factors

Studies have been made into the effects of infection, stress and trauma on MS. It is popularly believed that surgery and head injuries may accelerate the development of MS, as may stressful life events such as divorce, unemployment or moving house. A study that threw doubt on these factors precipitating MS did reveal an increase in respiratory, gastrointestinal and skin infections in the two weeks before an MS attack. Clearly research that provides information such as this may ultimately help in the management of MS.

Management and rehabilitation

Why must MS keep interfering with what I want to do in life? What can make life better for people with MS?

Since there is always the possibility that not only the frills but the basics of living well with MS will be eroded by the disease, vital research and testing are carried out to reduce the effects of MS symptoms and provide relief. While the cause of and cure for MS are still being searched for, everything that can be done to make life with MS easier is also being investigated. Although this type of research will not halt the disease process itself, quality of life with MS can be improved physically, emotionally, socially and at work. This is done firstly through psychosocial and rehabilitation research projects, and secondly, in a practical way, by working alongside people with MS and their families. Quality of life is of paramount importance. People with MS should always be involved in making an assessment of priorities, more particularly so when resources are limited. Coping with MS is an enormous task and requires detailed information and supportive back-up to be of any lasting benefit.

Rehabilitation is too often thought of as offering physical help only. But this is achieved most skilfully via a team approach in which each practitioner – the occupational therapist, pharmacologist, physiotherapist, surgeon or continence advisor – has a sensitive understanding of the psychology of living with a chronic disease.

One difficulty with any treatments that aid rehabilitation (from a scientific perspective at least) is how to evaluate the true results of trials. If the usefulness of physiotherapy or yoga is being tested, it is hard to give one group of people with MS real and a control group pretend yoga or physiotherapy. It is important not to overlook the fact that everyone is susceptible to the influence of suggestion. This is the so-called 'placebo effect', the improvement you feel if something is being done at all, regardless of what it is and how realistic it is to expect a positive outcome. With a disease like MS, emotional depression is relatively common, and so any ray of hope, improved support and an increase in activities and interests will do a lot to boost morale and make it appear to all concerned that real improvement has taken place, not only in spirits but neurologically too. It takes time and the discipline of double-blind testing to prove the basis for any apparent improvement.

From the perspective of people with MS, anything that might help is worth a try. MS can be so restricting that practical improvements now, no matter how apparently minor in terms of an ultimate cure, would be so freeing. These include remaining as comfortable and pain-free as possible, maintaining an optimal level of independence, being able to get to where we want to go – transport, access to all buildings, retraining for new jobs or pastimes and no discrimination because of MS – and therapies that enhance well-being physically, mentally, emotionally and spiritually. It makes a world of difference to people with MS and all who care for and about them that treatments like physiotherapy and services such as continence advice, sexual counselling, speech therapy and cognitive rehabilitation are readily available. It is a simple matter of human dignity: to be enabled to take responsibility and make a contribution.

Symptomatic treatments

Research and testing are also carried out to reduce the effects of MS symptoms and provide relief. Even if the disease process itself may not be altered, the quality of life with MS must be improved. Symptomatic treatments include a range of drugs and simple surgical procedures to correct any particular problems.

It is good that people with MS want to find ways of walking better or controlling their hand movements and that research into how this can be achieved is ongoing. Impaired movement can result for a number of different reasons: weak muscles, spasticity, loss of co-ordination, lack of balance and/or impaired sensation. Anti-spasmodic drugs, muscle relaxants or anti-inflammatory drugs along with physiotherapy and yoga are common and effective ways of helping people with MS to keep supple, co-ordinated and mobile. These approaches have been refined by the use of electronics to determine what causes muscle weakness. It can be due to actual weakness itself or the fact that the messages to the muscles are not getting through. Electronic muscle stimulation devices, together with appropriate exercises to make muscles work are found to be beneficial.

In a similar way the effect of drugs like beta-interferon can also be monitored. Beta-interferon is promising in the relapsing-remitting type of MS (see p. 105). It reduces the frequency of attacks and demyelination is visibly less evident on scans. Despite its expense, the inconvenience of the injections and side-effects, many people with MS welcome the possible long-term benefits of beta-interferon and immuno-modulating drugs and look forward to being able to maintain their independence as a result.

Other examples of symptomatic treatments include attempts to cope with weakness and fatigue and eliminate bladder and bowel disturbances. Remaining problems are the control of tremor, gait, sexual dysfunction, cognitive disturbance and some kinds of pain.

The previous chapter covers a number of currently popular symptomatic treatments.

Diet

There is clear evidence that nutrition can have profound effects on immune functions, resistance to infection and auto-immunity. Vitamins A and E, zinc and dietary lipids are especially important. There is additional evidence from other auto-immune diseases that the use of a low-fat diet and essential fatty acid supplements such as sunflower, the even richer safflower, borage and fungal oils are beneficial. Recent work by Laurence Harbige has focused on the fatty acids derived from linoleic acids in animal models of MS. The findings appear to show that linoleic acid reduces the severity of the animal form of the disease. Even more promising is the finding that the longer-chain fatty acids produced from the conversion of gamma-linolenic acids at specific doses apparently prevents the disease occurring at all in the animals. What is true for rats may hopefully prove true for people with MS.

Scientific controlled studies on diet and MS have concentrated on polyunsaturated fatty acids (PUFAs). PUFAs are important for growth and repair in nervous tissue and they also keep cell membranes fluid and flexible. In MS they help not only to maintain healthy tissue but ward off attack and can repair damage as well. These two specialized roles are vital to improvement in MS. It appears from animal models of MS that PUFAs work to protect the immune system and may also be the building blocks for the repair of myelin.

It is to be hoped that new tests on the effects of PUFAs, verified by MRI scans will soon be funded. Certainly many find improvement in their MS when they supplement their diets with PUFAs. The pattern of low levels of linoleic acid – a component of PUFAs – found in the serum of persons with MS, who also tend to have an unusual pattern of fatty acids in their blood, is reported to become normal within a year if a diet rich in PUFAs is followed. Certainly a diet rich in animal saturated fats reduces the biological effects of essential fatty acids. Thus a low saturated fat diet, rich in polyunsaturated acids, is considered the optimum diet to reduce the effect of MS. Linoleic acid has been shown to have a beneficial effect on the severity and duration of relapses and also slows down the progression of disability for those with early relapsing and remitting MS. It is thought likely that the combination of a low animal fat/high PUFA diet with supplementary linoleic acid is most beneficial for symptom and disease control.

Tissue bank donor card

Signing such a card gives the MS Society tissue bank permission to remove tissues (mainly from the brain and spinal cord), essential to research on MS after the donor dies. Analysis of such tissues will greatly help in developing new treatments and therapies for MS. There are MS tissue banks in London and Belfast.

Evaluating new therapies

Whatever new treatment, drug regime or therapy becomes popular and is greeted with hope and excitement, it is important that you know how to evaluate it, and also how researchers and the medical profession will make their evaluations.

You will need to consider whether any clinical improvement in your MS is a result of the therapy or would have happened anyway in the natural course of the disease. It is also necessary to keep in mind certain basic facts about neurological illness. One is that some neurological symptoms are rapidly reversible. Whether they appear or disappear seems to bear little relationship to demyelination; they can just as well be affected by temperature and fatigue, for example. It should also be borne in mind that some lesions are 'silent' – that is, they have no signs or symptoms. Thus any improvement in your MS may not be due in any way to a change in the lesions. In fact, any lesion that has become a dense scar is unlikely to improve, neither is any neurological dysfunction that has persisted for over two years. Also, sometimes certain medications prescribed to help MS problems have a physiological anti-depressant effect and this can make it difficult to assess how successful a new therapy really is.

In the end any therapy will stand or fall on the grounds of how beneficial it is to how many people, taking into account the risk to the taker and the cost in terms of money, time and effort.

USEFUL ADDRESSES

Organizations specializing in MS

The Multiple Sclerosis Society of Great Britain and Northern Ireland
Headquarters
25 Effie Road, Fulham, London SW6 1EE
Tel: 0171–610 7171
Fax: 0171–736 9861 or 0171–610 9912
Helpline: 0171–371 8000 (10am to 4pm Monday to Friday)
e-mail: Info@mssociety.org.uk
web site: http://www.mssociety.org.uk

The Multiple Sclerosis Society in Scotland
2a North Charlotte Street, Edinburgh EH2 4HR
Tel: 0131–225 3600

The Multiple Sclerosis Society Northern Ireland Office
34 Annadale Avenue, Belfast BT7 3JJ
Tel: 01232 644914

The Multiple Sclerosis Society Counselling Lines
(24-hour service via referral from answerphones listed below)
London 0171–222 3123
Midlands 0121–476 4229
Scotland 0131–226 6573

The MS Society offers advice and an information service by letter and phone (9am to 5pm). Its Helpline is staffed by advice workers offering an information service on MS. The MS Society also provides a network of over 360 local branches. It is the largest provider of funds for research into MS, these being administered through a medical research advisory committee. It also operates respite care and holiday centres, and publishes *MS Matters* (six times a year), and a range of informative publications free. It is a member of the International Federation of MS Societies (IFMSS).

linked together with careful attention being paid to breath control. Even if you are unable to move an arm or a leg, allowing yourself to visualize the movement you plan to make and then controlling the breath to give you energy while someone else lifts and moves the limb is also beneficial. It is often difficult with MS to move or hold a position, but just trying to do so often seems to have a retraining effect on the body. It is well worth overcoming any initial reluctance or desire to give up, if results are not immediate. Yoga seems to work like a key, unlocking resources in the body that help people live better with MS.

Yoga classes are quite popular. With MS you may find you can fit in easily enough with a regular class. Alternatively there are special remedial yoga classes designed specifically to help you overcome the disabilities of MS.

Aromatheraphy

Aromatherapists believe that essential oils, extracted from plants, can be absorbed through the skin. Once the oils have penetrated the skin, they are thought to travel to organs, glands and tissues and to seep into the bloodstream and lymph fluid of the body, the results of which may prove healing. Also the natural anti-bacterial and anti-viral properties of essential oils appear to increase resistance to infection.

Each essential oil has its own distinctive properties, which have an effect on both body and mind and also influence the emotions. Many oils seem to serve a multi-purpose function and it makes fascinating reading to discover which favour which part of the body.

By far the best and most effective way of using essential oils is in massage. The reaction of rubbing is thought to activate the nerve endings and stimulate the circulation of blood at the surface of the skin. In any case, a good massage is of itself relaxing and promotes a good sense of well-being. Essential oils can also be added to a warm bath. There they not only come in contact with the skin but are also inhaled.

Whether or not you accept the theory of aromatherapy, there can be no doubt that it is a most pleasant way of pampering yourself. Even if its beneficial results come solely from enjoying the scent of the oils, together with massage and baths, the psychological boost it gives invariably has a positive effect on health.

Biofeedback

This is a method of learning to become more aware of how the body responds and of finding beneficial ways of controlling its reactions. The principle behind it is that once you become aware of some body function, you can learn to control that function. It involves a certain degree of self-awareness, and employs the techniques of yoga as well as the technology of modern biofeedback machinery.

More preventative than curative, biofeedback seems to have some value for MS. This probably lies with the stress factor of MS. The ability to cope with stress depends on recognizing stress reactions in the body. Many people are never fully aware of effects of stress on their body and struggle on in a state of partial tension. By keeping the body under partial tension, they become prone to psychosomatic problems which may aggravate MS. Using a biofeedback machine that monitors electrical skin resistance can show them how to recognize body reactions to stress and warn them that they need to relax.

TENS (Transcutaneous Electrical Nerve Stimulation)

TENS is the application of a low-level pulse electrical current into the body through electrodes placed on the skin. This self-treatment unit is popular with people with MS as a means of reducing and even eliminating pain. The current apparently restricts the transmission of pain impulses while stimulating the body to produce its own pain-relieving hormones.

TENS units are widely used in hospitals and pain clinics and are gaining in popularity with physiotherapists. Small, lightweight and portable, they are easy to use and invaluable in the control of many of the pains that are associated with MS.

Hyperbaric oxygen (HBO)

One of the treatments some people with MS value is HBO. The term 'hyperbaric' means high pressure and HBO treatment consists of breathing in oxygen through a face mask while sitting in a metal chamber where the air pressure has been raised by pumping in oxygen. The theory behind the treatment is that oxygen at higher pressure can suppress inflammation around the MS diseased areas of the brain and prevent its spread. Those undergoing HBO treatment should not suffer from epilepsy or any heart condition.

In the early 1980s there was general excitement over sensational reports in the media of cures or considerable improvement as a result of HBO treatment. There was a rush for places and volunteers underwent training in the supervision of HBO chambers. Various trials to assess the true clinical value of HBO treatment have since overtiring yourself in a work-out which it takes days to recover from.

Physiotherapy treatment is normally arranged in Britain by your GP on an out-patient appointment basis. It can be both time-consuming and exhausting to wait for transport to and from out-patient clinics and this can counteract the benefit of the actual treatment. Occasionally, however, it is possible for a physiotherapist to come to your home to treat you. Physiotherapy is also available privately.

Massage

A good massage both relaxes and stimulates. General massage improves the circulation of the blood, thus aiding the nervous and immune systems to work at peak efficiency. Massage can also focus on relieving muscle tension and spasm. An old-fashioned technique called 'cupping' applied either side of the spinal cord has proved valuable for some people with MS. Massage works well in combination with bathing first. You must expect to feel very tired after it and may need time to build up a tolerance to its undoubtedly beneficial long-term effects.

Reflexology

More than just another form of massage, reflexology can be beneficial to people with MS. It is based on the principle of the body being divided into zones, each linked to a key point on one of the feet. By massaging the appropriate area of the foot, it is possible to treat the problems in the related body zone or organ. Simple and harmless, it often produces surprising results.

Yoga

Yoga will work successfully as long as you are willing to accept some of its philosophy as well as its practice. It is not a form of treatment, but more a way of taking control of yourself and making a conscious decision to integrate body, mind and spirit into a smoothly functioning whole. If you have time for the whole person approach and are sympathetic to the concept that good health depends on harmony, balance and maintaining natural rhythms, you will discover that yoga has much to offer.

Yoga seems to provide an antidote to the tensions of MS – both the tensions that arise as a consequence of the disease itself and those that are a reaction to living with it. There's no doubt that both types of tension can build up to such an extent that people easily

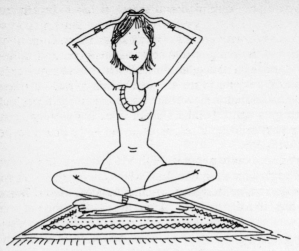

YOGA WILL WORK SUCCESSFULLY FOR YOU AS LONG
AS YOU ARE WILLING TO ACCEPT SOME OF ITS PHILOSOPHY
AS WELL AS ITS PRACTICE.

get locked into MS. Yoga counteracts this by allowing you to function fully once more, no longer fragmented but able to harness the total of what you are so that it is easier to cope. It invites you to accept life as it comes and teaches the skills to work in a systematic but relaxed way within the restrictions of the disease or problem area. It gives you a new option to choose in the place of grim determination and gritting your teeth when faced with a setback. Enthusiasts claim that yoga has much to offer that is of specific benefit to a disease like MS because it can maximize energy, give new tone to the neuromuscular system, have a positive effect on the immune system, improve the function of the glands, build up resistance to illness and keep the body supple.

Yoga teaches you how to breathe for maximum benefit so that tensions in your body are released and its energy is made fully available. The basis of energy control is knowing how to relax. During relaxation gentle diaphragmatic breathing maintains a continual flow of energy. In addition to this you need to practise specific breath control involving the diaphragm. By taking a strong breath in and then breathing out slowly, you are giving more oxygen to the body and brain and stimulating energy flow. This control of mind, body and energy is fully co-ordinated when you involve yoga movements, or asanas. Yoga movements can be done lying down, sitting on a chair or standing. Many are very simple, the more complex ones being a combination of simpler movements,

Tel: 01767 627271
They run a residential treatment centre with special weekend
courses and holidays, and train teachers to work with people
with disabilities, especially those with MS.

Organizations dealing with general disability and caring

Association of Crossroads Care Attendant Schemes Ltd
10 Regent Place, Rugby, Warwickshire, CV21 2PN
Tel: 01788 573653
24 George Square, Glasgow G2 1EG
Tel: 0141–226 3793
This scheme aims to relieve stress in the families or carers of
disabled people by offering domiciliary support services in local
areas.

Association of Disabled Professionals
170 Benton Hill, Wakefield Road, Horbury, W. Yorkshire, WF4
5HW
Tel: 01924 270335
A self-help group that focuses on support and advice in relation
to employment.

The BBC Helpline
Tel: 0800–044 044

British Association for Counselling
1 Regent Place, Rugby, Warwickshire, CV21 2PJ
Tel: 01788 550899
Fax: 01788 562189
Information line: 01788 578328

British Nursing Association
North Place, 82 Great North Road, Hatfield, Herts, AL9 5BL
Tel: 017072 63544

British Red Cross Society
9 Grosvenor Crescent, London SW1X 7EJ
Tel: 0171–235 6315

Carers National Association
Ruth Pitter House, 20–25 Glasshouse Yard, London EC1A 4JS
Tel: 0171–490 8818
Fax: 0171–490 8824
Carers' Line: 0171–490 8898
This is the leading voluntary organization working to advise
carers and encourage them to recognize their own needs. CNA

promotes the interests of carers within government and other policy makers.

Citizens' Advice, Scotland
26 George Square, Edinburgh EH8 9LD
Tel: 0131–667 0156

The Continence Foundation
Basement, 2 Doughty Street, London WC1N 2PH
Tel: 0191–213 0050 (Helpline: 9am–6pm)

Dial UK (National Association of Disablement Information and Advice Lines)
Park Lodge, St Catherine's Hospital, Tickhill Road, Balby, Doncaster, S. Yorkshire. DN4 8QN
Tel: 01302 310123
An autonomous association of people with personal experience of disability with the primary aim of providing a comprehensive and confidential information and advice service on any matter relating to disability. They liaise with over 100 local offices nationwide.

The Disability Alliance
First Floor East, Universal House, 88–94 Wentworth Street, London E1 7SA
Tel: 0171–247 8776
Rights Advice Line: (3 sessions per week) 0171–247 8763 (on Minicom)
The Disability Alliance offers a 'rights service' by telephone, publishes the invaluable Disability Rights Handbook and other publications on benefit and aims to introduce a comprehensive income scheme for disabled people.

Disability Law Service
16 Princeton Street, London WC1R 4BB
Tel: 0171–831 8031/7740
It provides a broad range of legal advice and assistance for people with a disability and their families. Advice is given by telephone and correspondence, and a solicitor will see you by appointment.

Disabled Drivers Association
Ashwellthorpe Hall, Ashwellthorpe, Norwich, NR16 1EX
Tel: 01508 489449

Disabled Drivers Insurance Bureau
292 Hale Lane, Edgware, Middlesex, HA8 8NP
Tel: 0181–958 3135

The Disabled Living Foundation
380–384 Harrow Road, London W9 2HU
Tel: 0171–289 6111
They provide information and advice on daily living equipment
for people with a disability.

Disablement Income Group (DIG)
Millmead Business Centre, Millmead Road, London N17 9QU
Tel: 0171–263 3981
DIG's aim is to promote the financial welfare of disabled people
through a programme of advice, advocacy, field work,
information, public research and training.

Home Care Support
382 Hillcross Avenue, Morden, Surrey, SM4 4EX
Tel: 0181–542 0348

Kings Fund Centre
11–13 Cavendish Square, London W1M 0AN
Tel: 0171–307 2400
The centre is a policy advisory body that researches into the
information and support helpful to people with different
conditions and to those supporting them.

Leonard Cheshire Foundation
26–29 Maunsel Street, London SE1P 2QN
Tel: 0171–828 1822

Mobility Advice and Insurance Service (MAVIS)
Transport and Road Research Laboratory, Old Wokingham Road,
Crowthorne, Berkshire, RG11 6AU
Tel: 01344 770456

Mobility Information Service
Unit 2A, Atcham Estate, Shrewsbury, SY4 4UG
Tel: 01743 761889

Motability
2nd Floor, Gate House, West Gate, The High, Harlow, Essex,
CM20 1HR
Tel: 01279 635666
Motability is a registered charity which helps people to use their
mobility allowance to lease a new car or buy a new car, scooter
or wheelchair on credit terms.

The National Association of Citizens' Advice Bureaux
Middleton House, 115–123 Pentonville Road, London N1 9LZ
Tel: 0171–251 2000

The Open University – Advisor to Disabled Students
Walton Hall, Milton Keynes, MK7 6AA
Tel: 01908 653442

Opportunities for People with Disabilities
1 Bank Buildings, Princes Street, London EC2R 8EU
Tel: 0171–726 4961 and 0171–726 4963 (Minicom)
Opportunities aims through training, preparation and guidance
to help people with disabilities find jobs matched to their talents
and aspirations by persuading employers to positively recognize
abilities and potentials.

PHAB (Physically Handicapped and Able-Bodied)
12–14 London Road, Croydon, CR0 2TA
Tel: 0181–667 9443
PHAB seeks to achieve the integration of able-bodied and
disabled people in all aspects of life.

RELATE National Marriage Guidance
Herbert Gray College, Little Church Street, Rugby, CV21 3AP
Tel: 01788 573241

**The Royal Association for Disability and Rehabilitation
(RADAR)**
12 City Forum, 250 City Road, London EC1V 8AF
Tel: 0171–250 3222
RADAR acts as a pressure group, locally and nationally, to
improve life for physically disabled people. It provides
comprehensive information on disability issues such as access,
education, employment, housing, holidays, mobility and benefits.
It is responsible for the administration of the National Key
Scheme for access to adapted public toilets.

SKILL – National Bureau for Students with Disabilities
Tel: 0171–978 9890

**SPOD – Association to Aid the Sexual and Personal
Relationships of People with a Disability**
286 Camden Road, London N7 0BJ
Tel: 0171–607 8851/2
SPOD offers information, general leaflets and a reading list. It
also operates a counselling line.

Further Reading

Learning to Live with Multiple Sclerosis R. Povey, R. Dowey and G. Prett (Sheldon Press)

Living with MS Elizabeth Forsythe, MRCS LRCP DPH (Faber and Faber)

McAlpine's Multiple Sclerosis Edited by W. B. Matthews (Longman Group UK Ltd)

Multiple Sclerosis – A Personal Exploration Alexander Burnfield (Souvenir Press)

Multiple Sclerosis – A Self-Help Guide to its Management Judy Graham (B. H. Blackwell Ltd)

Multiple Sclerosis – Exploring Sickness and Health Elizabeth Forsythe, MRCS LRCP DPH (Faber and Faber)

Multiple Sclerosis – Psychological and Social Aspects Edited by Aart Simons (Heinemann Medical Books)

Multiple Sclerosis – The Facts W. B. Matthews, DM FRCP (Oxford University Press)

Standing in the Sunshine: The Story of the MS Breakthrough Cari Loder (Century Press)

Symptom Management in Multiple Sclerosis Randall Schapiro (Costello)

The Multiple Sclerosis Fact Book Richard Lechtenberg (Waverley Europe)

Therapeutic Claims in Multiple Sclerosis William Sibley (John Smith and Son, Glasgow University Bookshop [Tel: 0141–339 1463])

You and Caring – An Action Plan for Caring at Home Penny Mares (Kings Fund Centre)

INDEX